CATCHING CANCER

CATCHING CANCER

The Quest for Its Viral and Bacterial Causes

Claudia Cornwall

ROWMAN & LITTLEFIELD PUBLISHERS, INC.
Lanham • Boulder • New York • Toronto • Plymouth, UK

Published by Rowman & Littlefield Publishers, Inc.
A wholly owned subsidiary of The Rowman & Littlefield Publishing Group, Inc.
4501 Forbes Boulevard, Suite 200, Lanham, Maryland 20706
www.rowman.com

10 Thornbury Road, Plymouth PL6 7PP, United Kingdom

British Library Cataloguing in Publication Information Available

Library of Congress Cataloging-in-Publication Data

Cornwall, Claudia Maria.
Catching cancer : the quest for its viral and bacterial causes / Claudia Cornwall.
p. ; cm.
Includes bibliographical references.
ISBN 978-1-4422-1520-7 (cloth : alk. paper) -- ISBN 978-1-4422-1522-1 (electronic)
I. Title. [DNLM: 1. Neoplasms--history. 2. Neoplasms--microbiology. 3. History, 20th Century. 4. Oncogenic Viruses--pathogenicity. QZ 11.1]
616.99'4--dc23
2012044457

™ The paper used in this publication meets the minimum requirements of American National Standard for Information Sciences Permanence of Paper for Printed Library Materials, ANSI/NISO Z39.48-1992.

Printed in the United States of America

They are the taboo breakers who enjoy the whiff of grapeshot and the crackle of thin ice. —E. O. Wilson

CONTENTS

ACKNOWLEDGMENTS

Many people helped me to write this book. I would like to thank my husband, Gordon Cornwall, who has supported me in so many ways, perhaps most of all by insisting that I carry on with the project, despite his serious medical issues. Palmer Beasley, Lu-Yu Hwang, and Cladd Stevens were generous with their recollections of their research in Taiwan. Bruce Beasley told me stories about his brother's childhood. Harvey Alter and Timothy Block contributed their insights about the history of hepatitis B research. Tiffany Shih found and translated relevant newspaper articles, and Tilman Aretz clarified the mysterious world of Taiwan's officialdom for me. I'd like to thank Harald zur Hausen and his colleagues for giving me so much of their time: Heinrich Schulte-Holthausen, Matthias Dürst, Michael Boshart, Elisabeth Schwarz, Lutz Gissman, and Magnus von Knebel-Doeberitz. I'd also like to thank Manfred and Winfried zur Hausen for their memories. Bernard Roizman, George Klein, Clyde Goodheart, and Andre Nahmias helped me to re-create a fateful meeting in Key Biscayne. Barry Marshall and Robin Warren gave me long interviews, and John Papadimitriou, Arthur Morris, David Foreman, and Martin Skirrow all took me back to the early days of *H. pylori* research. Paul Ewald gave me several hours of his time, and Patrick Moore was patient with my many questions. Robert Holt helped me to see some of the new directions the research was taking. Kristine Fersovich and Arline kindly gave me the patient's point of view. I'd like to thank the Canadian Institutes for Health Research for the initial grant which helped get the book off the ground and also my editors at *Reader's Digest Canada*, Mary Aikins and Peter Stockland, for accepting my proposal to write an article about cancer and infections—my first foray into the topic. Finally, I'd like to acknowledge my agent, Robert Lecker, and my editor, Suzanne Staszak-Silva, for their enthusiasm and encouragement.

INTRODUCTION

In the Face of General Opinion

"Have they got a cure yet?" the cabby asked, looking inquiringly at me in the rearview mirror. We'd been chatting, and he'd wanted to know what brought me to Toronto. I told him I'd come to hear some lectures about cancer. Like everyone else, my driver was aware that for years, researchers had been seeking a cure. When people thought about vanquishing cancer, this naturally came to mind. I said that scientists were working toward *preventing* the disease. If they succeeded, millions of people would never get sick, would never need a cure. He smiled at me. I wasn't sure whether he approved or was skeptical and too polite to say anything.

It was November 2009, and I was attending a conference at the University of Toronto to commemorate the fiftieth anniversary of the Canadian Gairdner Awards. Researchers from all around the world have won these prizes for (among other things) eradicating smallpox, curing ulcers, inventing CT scans, and creating immune-suppressing drugs that make organ transplants possible. The three-day event was a celebration of discovery. Winners from previous years came to join in the festivities, and because many of them had gone on to win the Nobel Prize, it was a star-studded assembly indeed.

Students, professors, members of the public, and journalists like me listened in on the sessions held under the domed rotunda in Convocation Hall. Scientists spoke about stem cells, the challenge of chronic disease, the immune system, infections, and cancer. I remember one panel discussion about the possibility of sequencing one's own genome. Dr. Michael Hayden, a renowned geneticist (who identified the genes responsible for Huntington's disease and other disorders), moderated the conversation. When he invited questions from the audience, a hushed silence descended. He said, "You know, you don't *have* to be a Nobel Prize–winner to ask a question." A few shy hands went up.

I was interested in the lectures about cancer and infection because I was gathering research material for a magazine article. When Dr. Harald zur Hausen began to speak, I paid particular attention. The previous year, he had won a Nobel Prize for the discovery that the human papillomavirus (HPV) causes cervical cancer, a disease which kills 275,000 women every year. The world's third most common cancer in women, it exacts a grave toll, especially in developing countries that have few screening programs and limited treatment options. Zur Hausen's research made possible a vaccine that prevents 70 percent of cervical cancers. By 2009, Merck & Co., the pharmaceutical company making it, had dispensed 40 million doses.

A courtly, dignified man in his early seventies, zur Hausen spoke quietly and precisely. He made few hand gestures and eschewed rhetorical flourishes, but his story was dramatic. He said that globally, 21 percent of cancers (over 2.5 million cases annually) were now linked to infections. This was quite a shift from just forty years earlier, when scientists had not identified a single infectious cause of a human cancer. Moreover, we now had vaccines—to prevent cervical *and* liver cancer. Zur Hausen expressed his confidence that more breakthroughs would follow. He noted that in the past fifteen years, investigators had found several suspicious viruses and virus families.

As I sat on my hard wooden chair listening to zur Hausen and watching the numbers and graphs scroll behind him on the screen, I wondered if this is what a medical revolution felt like. Cancer was one of the most feared of all sicknesses, known since ancient times. At home, I had a book called *The Dread Disease*.[1] A history of the illness, it described how cancerphobia is deeply rooted in American culture. Would our apprehensions about it be lessening now? Was a new era beginning?

Like other major shifts in thinking, this one had taken time to get rolling. I knew that zur Hausen ran into strenuous opposition at first. The Nobel Prize Committee commended him for going "against current dogma" and said his suggestions "flew in the face of general opinion." Curious about that, I went down to the front of the auditorium after his talk and introduced myself. He graciously shook my hand, and when I asked him what gave rise to his ideas, he told me that since the 1930s scientists had known viruses caused cancer in animals. He believed they were also responsible for some of the disease in humans. Few researchers agreed with him though. He recalled that "very eminent" scientists scoffed at these notions. "They said, 'We know what causes cancer and it isn't viruses.'" And then he smiled broadly.

The next speaker was Dr. Barry Marshall, an extroverted Australian, who together with his colleague, Dr. Robin Warren, won the Nobel in 2005 for the discovery that a corkscrew-shaped bacterium called *Helicobacter pylori* (or *H. pylori*) induced gastritis, an inflammation of the stomach lining, as well as stomach ulcers. These conditions often led to stomach cancer, a major killer globally, responsible for 800,000 deaths a year. It was the second deadliest cancer. (Lung cancer is responsible for the most deaths.) *H. pylori* was the bacterium that wasn't supposed to be there. When Warren and Marshall embarked on their journey of inquiry, the consensus was that *no* bacteria could survive in stomach acid—equal in strength to car battery acid. The two doctors had a hard time persuading their medical colleagues that the bacteria even existed. Once they grudgingly conceded this point, the next hurdle for the Australian physicians was persuading their peers that the bacteria *caused* gastritis and peptic ulcers. This too was contrary to mainstream opinion, which blamed stress, smoking, and eating spicy foods. One popular rebuttal of Marshall's account of the situation was to say that gastritis and ulcers came first, creating favorable conditions for the bacteria which opportunistically followed.

Marshall said that he couldn't experiment on animals to show that the bacteria created stomach difficulties. Apparently animals didn't react the same way we did to *H. pylori*. Then Marshall hit upon a daring solution—a way to break the conceptual log jam. He drank a cocktail of *H. pylori* himself and documented what happened. On the screen behind him, he pointed at the historic slide of his own stomach with the *H. pylori* taking hold on the tenth day after he swallowed his bug broth. The germs produced an acute gastritis. Marshall felt violently ill and vomited. This was just the proof he needed. It was clear: the microbes *preceded* the inflammation. Marshall had to do more work to persuade the medical establishment that he was right. But his demonstration was the tipping point. Patients around the world heard about it and began asking their doctors to put them on the radical new cure for ulcers that an Australian physician was advocating—antibiotics. Marshall went on to explain that *H. pylori* was a complicated bacterium. For one thing, it came in different strains. Asia had high rates of stomach cancer because the *H. pylori* varieties prevalent there were particularly virulent. Marshall concluded by saying that researchers were trying to develop a vaccine, but in the meantime, antibiotics could be used to treat *H. pylori* infections.

As Marshall spoke, I saw that both he and zur Hausen wanted to change our view of cancer substantially. For years, we've blamed lifestyle choices (diet, smoking, lack of exercise, alcohol), environmental factors (ultraviolet rays, radiation, chemical toxins), and genetic inheritance for the disease. But these two scientists were saying that foreign pathogens should be added to the list of culprits. That meant our anticancer arsenal was suddenly larger and included vaccines, antivirals, and antibiotics. Since HPV is sexually transmitted, even condoms were a weapon in this fight (although they don't offer perfect protection against HPV). While it is not entirely clear how *H. pylori* travels from one host to another, some suspect contaminated food and water may transmit it. Thus, we might consider a program to clean up the water supply in communities where *H. pylori* is endemic.

Marshall's lecture also illustrated the power of theory—its iron grip—how it could even induce people not to see what was plainly before their eyes. This subject intrigued me too, and as I walked back to my hotel in the autumn rain, I thought I could really get my teeth into the topic. I wanted to know how medical theories changed. What kind of person was able to bring that about? How did revolutionaries endure the denial, the incredulity, perhaps even the ridicule that greeted a new idea? How could they press forward for years without much encouragement?

I flew back to my home in North Vancouver and began working on an article for *Reader's Digest Canada*, a magazine to which I had contributed for many years. I arranged to interview Harald zur Hausen by phone at his office in Heidelberg, Germany, and Barry Marshall by phone at his in Perth, Australia. I talked to Dr. Palmer Beasley in Houston, a man whose work on liver cancer made him part of this pioneering triumvirate. Liver cancer is also a major disease, killing 700,000 people worldwide every year—our third most common cancer. Like zur Hausen and Marshall, Beasley faced skepticism. When he started a study to investigate whether the virus responsible for hepatitis B also caused liver cancer, he said, "I was told to stop it." He recalled that some of his peers thought "I was really barking up the wrong tree."

I also talked to people who were personally affected by these advances in medical practice. I spoke to Kristine Fersovich, an Edmonton mother who had been diagnosed with cervical cancer when she was twenty-eight and who had surgery to treat it. Her mother had the same disease at the same age and, like Fersovich, was successfully treated. But Fersovich wanted to be sure her nine-year-old daughter didn't have to go through what she and her mother had experienced. She was keen to see her get the vaccine against HPV as soon as she was eligible to have it. I talked to some of the residents of Aklavik, a small village in northern Canada. They were concerned about the effects of *H. pylori* infection, and Dr. Karen Goodman, an epidemiologist at the University of Alberta, was working with them to see if she could help. She tested the villagers and began a pilot project to determine whether antibiotics—given to people who were positive for *H. pylori*—could prevent some of the problems associated with the bacteria. Dr. Goodman wanted to know what kinds of antibiotics performed best and how patients who were cured of *H. pylori* might avoid becoming re-infected. This was the new knowledge in action.

Reader's Digest Canada published my article in July 2010 under the title "Can You Catch Cancer?" But there was more to this topic than I could write in just a few pages. I wanted to delve deeper into the research and find out about some of the technical innovations and the scientific progress that created this revolution. Who were the people involved? Why did they succeed? What forces were arrayed against them? I wanted to visit some of the researchers in person, and explore the subject in a larger work. I began a book. I decided to call it "Catching Cancer" for two reasons. It would explain how several cancers were "caught" or understood, their mechanism laid bare. It would also be an account of the idea that you could "catch" some kinds of cancer, pick them up because of infections.

1

MORE THAN A CURIOSITY

. . . nature often speaks her secrets with a still, small voice out of a thicket of happenings.

—Francis Peyton Rous[1]

Distressed about a mysterious illness affecting his prize-winning fowl, a chicken farmer decided to consult experts at the Rockefeller Institute of Medical Research in New York (now Rockefeller University). It was 1909, and the institute was one of America's premier research facilities. Why did the breeder think such a prestigious organization was the right place to take his chicken? History is mute on this question. But we are all the richer for his dedicated husbandry. He was the man who drew back the curtain for the scientists, exposing a new vista for them to explore.

The farmer made his way from Long Island to Manhattan and arrived at the Rockefeller Institute with a barred Plymouth Rock hen tucked under his arm. She had a nasty growth on her breast, but only one researcher took an interest. That was Dr. Frances Peyton Rous, a newly minted physician, who had arrived at the institute just a few months before. He had agreed to take charge of cancer research there despite a warning from his mentor, Dr. William Welch, a professor at Johns Hopkins medical school. Welch thought cancer was a field in which it was too difficult to make progress. Rous, however, approached the challenge with all the enthusiasm of a young man wanting to make his mark in the world.

Unfortunately, the farmer's faith in the institute was not rewarded. Rous did not cure the bird, but his experiments quickly revealed a surprising fact about her tumor. Rous had a passion for experimental pathology, both for the chance it offered to discover something really new and for the discipline of careful observation that it imposed. One of his mantras was "Stay as close to nature as you can."[2] Rous recognized right away that the chicken had a malignant tumor that was given to widespread metastasis. To learn more about it, he extracted some cells and injected them into healthy chickens. They too became ill. In her study of his discovery, Eva Becsei-Kilborn explained, "All his experimentations on the chicken sarcoma seemed to suggest that it was the cells themselves from which the cancerous growths originated."[3] But Peyton Rous decided to go one step further. He wondered whether it was really the malignant cells that transmitted the cancer—or something else.

He had a possible suspect in mind, a kind of pathogen that had recently been identified. Too tiny to be seen in microscopes of the day, it could nevertheless be extracted from animal or plant tissue and its effects studied. Scientists had learned these agents were associated with highly contagious diseases. Today we know them as viruses, but at the time researchers did not understand them very well. They had not finally settled whether they were living organisms or chemical stimulants of some kind. According to Becsei-Kilborn, nothing in Rous's previous research indicated that such novel entities might be the culprits. It was a leap—a lucky hunch.

The new kind of pathogen could be separated from larger entities such as bacteria and other cells with a filter. To find out whether it was present in the chicken tumor, Peyton Rous ground it up and suspended it in a special salt solution. Then he passed the broth through progressively finer filters to hold back the malignant cells. When he injected the liquid that had passed through the filters into a healthy chicken, it developed the same tumor the diseased chicken had. He wrote that then "the host rapidly emaciates, becomes cold, somnolent, and dies."[4] As Becsei-Kilborn explained, "This indicated that something had been separated from the malignant cell which was so small that it could not be seen with the microscope and yet was capable of reproducing the cancerous tumor. This was of considerable significance because, for

Rous, it meant that an ultramicroscopic agent was the underlying cause of the chicken sarcoma."[5]

Peyton Rous published an article about his intriguing finding in 1911 and received a Nobel Prize for the discovery, decades later in 1966, when he was eighty-six years old. Although he had to wait an exceedingly long time before being recognized with the coveted award, Becsei-Kilborn points out that his work was not exactly ignored at the time. However, the majority of researchers were not convinced that Rous had found something which could help to explain human cancers. For one thing, although he tried for two years to find something similar in rats and mice, he was unable to do so. This lent credence to the idea that what Rous uncovered was an anomaly. As Becsei-Kilborn recounts, this was how people like E. E. Tyzzer, chairman of the Harvard University Cancer Commission, understood the matter: "Notwithstanding the interest which the work on fowl tumors aroused, in no instance has a similar infectious agent been demonstrated in tumors of mammals. We have at present, then, no grounds for believing that here is any specific infection associated with human tumors."[6]

In the late nineteenth century, encouraged by the successes of scientists like Louis Pasteur and Robert Koch, researchers began to look for microbial causes of cancer. But by the early twentieth century, all promising leads seemed to have dried up. The thinking shifted to the idea that cancer was probably the result of a cell's internal disorganization. Furthermore, Peyton Rous's proposal that cancer was caused by an infectious agent appeared to fly in the face of everyday observations. Becsei-Kilborn wrote, "Clinicians and surgeons were particularly critical of the infectious theory of cancer. Clinical experience showed that cancer was not contagious in person to person contacts. There were no reports of nurses, clinicians, or pathologists who came into close contact with the disease having been infected."[7] The "extrinsic" theory of cancer causation which blamed a foreign pathogen was losing out. The "intrinsic" hypothesis which maintained that cancer was essentially a breakdown in the machinery of the cell was gaining ground.

The tumor that Peyton Rous found was named after him, but in 1915, he left cancer research behind. In his own words: "I'd become pinched and parched mentally as a result of continually negative experimentation, and felt that only new outlooks could cure." Rous had an "urgent desire to escape from the thickening cloud of [my] ignorance."[8]

He entered a new field—blood physiology—and, in 1917, helped to establish the world's first blood bank in Belgium near the front lines of the First World War.

The idea that an infection of some kind was to blame for cancer did not die, but grew by fits and starts. The clues were scattered; researchers working in Africa, Asia, Australia, North America, and Europe all found pieces of the puzzle. It always seemed that progress came because a scientist noticed some small aberration from the ordinary. In the 1930s, a colleague of Rous's at Rockefeller, a veterinarian called Dr. Richard Shope, became interested in cottontail rabbits in the American southwest. They occasionally produced long horn-like growths on their heads. (These rabbits inspired stories about a creature called a Jackalope—a rabbit-antelope cross. The town of Douglas, Wyoming, still pays homage to those tall tales with the world's largest statue of the legendary animal—an eighty-foot sculpture.) Shope determined that a virus caused the "horns." Then, knowing of Rous's earlier interest in virus-induced cancers, he passed the growths on to him. Rous confirmed that they were a benign cancer. This was the first indication that viruses could cause a cancer in a mammal.

In 1936, Dr. John Bittner, a biologist at the Jackson Laboratory in Bar Harbor, Maine, found that a tendency to breast cancer in certain strains of mice could be transmitted from mothers to foster children. In other words, the offspring got it from their mothers, but not as part of their genetic inheritance. Bittner suspected that the mothers might be infecting the infant mice with a cancer-causing virus when they suckled. Cautiously, he called it a "milk factor." However, by 1946, he was confident he had found a virus and said so to a journalist at *Time*.[9] In 1951, Ludwik Gross, an Austrian-born physician working at the Bronx Veterans Administration Hospital in New York, proved that another virus passed from a mother to her offspring caused leukemia in mice.

Gross thought it was only a matter of time before investigators discovered a virus that caused the same cancer in humans. He wrote, "The various forms of leukemia developing in mice and in man are so similar in their clinical course, and morphology, that it would be quite difficult to assume that leukemia in humans is a disease fundamentally different from that observed in mice."[10] The view that the discoveries of Rous, Shope, Bittner, Gross, and others had wider implications was growing increasingly plausible. Yet the prize continued to elude scientists.

A breakthrough finally came, but not in one of the world's most important medical centers. It surfaced far away from the mainstream—in Africa. Denis Burkitt, an idealistic Irish doctor, was working in Mulago Hospital in Kampala, Uganda, in 1957, when he treated a five-year-old boy who had a massive swelling on his face. He had never seen anything like it. Shortly afterward, Dr. Burkitt saw another young patient affected the same way. He decided to investigate further because, as he wrote: "A curiosity can occur once, but two cases indicated more than a curiosity."[11] He found that the children were afflicted with a type of lymphoma, a cancer of the immune system. As soon as he recognized that, he saw that it was the most common childhood tumor in the area where he worked. When he consulted records at the oldest hospital in east Africa, the Mengo Mission Hospital in Kampala, he realized that this unusual disease was not new. He also noted that most cases seemed to come from the northeastern part of the country. When a South African pathologist and epidemiologist, Dr. George Oettle, told him that the condition was unknown in his home country, Burkitt surmised that it had something to do with geographic location.

Using a modest government grant totaling £25 to cover the cost of printing and mailing, Burkitt sent letters to hospitals and missions all across Africa, asking about the tumor. Burkitt's intuition was acute. It turned out that a "lymphoma belt" stretched across the middle of the continent from Kenya and Tanganika in the east to Dakar in the west. The disease was most prevalent in low-lying, moist, warm areas. In 1958, he published his first paper about the condition, but it attracted no attention whatsoever.

Then in March 1961, while in England on leave, Burkitt visited London and spoke about his work. An unknown doctor with a practice far removed from a famous university or institution, he did not attract large audiences. Only twelve people attended one of his talks, in a hall at the Royal College of Surgeons.[12] He might have been completely ignored were it not for one man who did hear him, and who was riveted—Dr. Anthony Epstein, a pathologist at Middlesex Hospital in London. He had studied Rous's sarcoma virus for a few years—one of a small coterie of researchers who appreciated that viruses could cause cancer. As he listened to Burkitt, he thought that this particular lymphoma might be a good candidate for that explanation. He was keen to investigate the tumor for unusual viruses, and when he approached Burkitt, the doctor agreed to send him samples.

Upon his return to Africa, Burkitt went on what he called a "tumor safari." He wanted to see the swath the disease was cutting through the continent and map its path, particularly its rather indistinct southern border. He wrote that it was to be something like a "geographical biopsy."[13] As he observed dryly, "This form of investigation, touring the African bush in a Ford station wagon that had already seen eight years of service in the Congo, is foreign to accepted concepts of cancer research, but has nevertheless proved fruitful."[14] In October 1961, he and two friends, both mission doctors, covered more than 10,000 miles over a period of ten weeks. They visited sixty hospitals in nine countries. The trek confirmed what Burkitt's correspondence with African hospitals seemed to reveal. Climate was key. The disease which came to be called Burkitt's lymphoma wasn't a problem where the yearly mean temperature was below 15 degrees Centigrade and where the annual rainfall was less than 20 inches. The dependence on climate showed that a biological organism of some kind was involved. In discussions with his colleagues the idea came up that it might be a virus. "We knew that certain animal tumors were virus-induced. Why not those in man?" Burkitt wrote.[15]

In the meantime, flights from Kampala started bringing regular deliveries of biopsies to London for Epstein to analyze. Over a period of two years, Epstein received a steady supply of lymphoma biopsies, and he and his research assistants, Yvonne Barr and Bert Achong, worked hard to find a virus using a variety of methods. All the results were negative until December 5, 1963, when a fortuitous accident occurred. The plane bearing Epstein's delivery was delayed by fog. When he got his sample, he discovered that the fluid in which the biopsy tissue was suspended was unusually cloudy. At first, he thought it was probably contaminated by bacteria. However, when he peered at it through a conventional light microscope, he saw that the cloudiness was due to a large number of individual tumor cells shaken loose from the tissue during the uncommonly long trip. Epstein succeeded in culturing these cells. Later he wrote that when he first inspected them with an electron microscope on February 24, 1964, he was "exhilarated to observe unequivocal virus particles."[16] A latent virus was activated.

This wasn't the end of the research on the lymphoma, though—a puzzling, elusive disease. Eventually, it seemed that the virus Epstein had discovered only caused the lymphoma in areas intensely affected by malaria. To this day, the relationship between Burkitt's lymphoma and malaria is not entirely understood, but the suspicion is that children whose immune systems are weakened by malaria are unable to ward off the virus and are at risk for cancer.

Did Epstein's discovery take the world by storm? Well, not exactly. Epstein wrote, "The climate of opinion at the time of the discovery was generally unsympathetic to the idea that viruses might play a role in human cancer causation. Thus, the recognition of EBV [Epstein-Barr virus, as it was eventually called] as a possible human tumor virus, even if only in the case of BL [Burkitt's lymphoma], took very much longer and only began very slowly once a great body of information had been built up on it."[17]

The hypothesis that dangerous chemicals were one of the main causes of cancer had become fashionable, both with scientists and the public. The famous report that Dr. Luther Terry, the US surgeon general, tabled on January 11, 1964, probably had a lot to do with that. On a Saturday (the day was chosen to reduce the impact on the stock market), he briefed two hundred reporters for two hours in a media lockup. The security measure was deemed necessary because Dr. Terry's brown book called "Smoking and Health" was so controversial. The report said that smokers were ten to twenty times more likely to develop lung cancer than nonsmokers. Later Dr. Terry recalled, "The report hit the country like a bombshell. It was front page news and a lead story on every radio and television station in the United States and many abroad. The report not only carried a strong condemnation of tobacco usage, especially cigarette smoking, but conveyed its message in such clear and concise language that it could not be misunderstood."[18] At that time, 46 percent of all Americans smoked. Within three months of Terry's report, cigarette consumption had dropped 20 percent. Although sales soon rebounded, tobacco continued to be assailed as a major health hazard.

Dr. Palmer Beasley recalled the viewpoint vividly. In an interview, he told me:

> It is true that some chemicals are highly carcinogenic and it is true that cigarettes, when smoked, are a terrible problem and I'm not trying to diminish that at all. Unfortunately, though, the National Cancer Institute and the country turned its back on its own history that had made essential earlier contributions in viral studies. They closed viral labs and said, "We're doing chemicals." They overdid it. In the process of looking for chemical causes, of which there aren't so many, and which aren't as important as they thought, they stopped thinking that viruses played important role in carcinogenesis. President Richard Nixon signed the National Cancer Act in 1971, starting the war on cancer. But it wasn't a war on cancer, it was a war on viruses.

What Beasley called the "war on viruses" was really an attack on the science which implicated viruses as causes of cancer. Eventually, it lost ground. Serendipity played a role, but equally important were the sage intuitions of a few scientists who took advantage of serendipitous observations. Louis Pasteur famously said, "Chance only favors the mind which is prepared." The remark, which was part of his inaugural address at the opening of the Faculté des Sciences at the University of Lille on December 7, 1854, is often quoted (and sometimes misquoted). I think it is worth putting it in context because of a couple other points that Pasteur made:

> Without theory, practice is but routine born of habit. Theory alone can bring forth and develop the spirit of invention. It is to you specially that it will belong not to share the opinion of those narrow minds who disdain everything in science which has not immediate application. You know [Benjamin] Franklin's charming saying? He was witnessing the first demonstration of a purely scientific discovery, and people round him said: "But what is the use of it?" Franklin answered them: "What is the use of a new-born child?". . .
> Do you know when this electric telegraph, one of the most marvelous applications of modern science, first saw the light? It was in the memorable year 1822; [Hans Christian] Oersted, a Danish physicist, held in his hands a piece of copper wire, joined by its extremities to the two poles of a Volta pile. On his table was a magnetized needle on its pivot, and he suddenly saw (by chance you will say, but chance favors only the mind which is prepared) the needle move and take up a position quite different from the one assigned to it by terrestrial

> magnetism. A wire carrying an electric current deviated a magnetized needle from its position! That, gentlemen, was the birth of the modern telegraph. Franklin's interlocutor might well have said when the needle moved: "But what is the use of that?" And yet that discovery was barely twenty years old when it produced by its application the almost supernatural effects of the electric telegraph![19]

Succinctly, Pasteur touched on three pillars of discovery. While science often gives rise to spectacular technological achievements, investigators need to be able to follow lines of inquiry whose immediate and useful application is not obvious. Those "gee whiz" results (the telegraph in Pasteur's day, the iPad in ours) ultimately rest on a deep understanding of nature's secrets. Secondly, theory gives rise to hypotheses and drives invention. It guides experimentation. Of course, false theories can lead us down blind allies sometimes, but learning that an alley is blind is also progress. Finally, the researcher makes many observations, but he or she needs to know what to do with them. Are they worth investigating further? If they are unexpected, is this mere "noise" or indicative of something new and important? Pasteur stressed the significance of the "prepared" mind. He didn't explain what that was, though. And as you will see in the stories that follow, preparation seems to take many different forms. We are not likely to find a formula that will tell us how to produce a brilliant scientist or a remarkable insight. But there are hints about some of the ingredients that may be necessary.

We often think of a "revolution" as a sudden and dramatic change. But this shift in medical thinking was gradual, about a hundred years in the making, with several important milestones along the way. The discovery that a virus helped cause Burkitt's lymphoma was important even though in global terms, only a small percentage of individuals were affected by the disease. This was the first time a human cancer could be linked to a virus. When zur Hausen showed that some human papillomaviruses caused cervical cancer, he also explained exactly how it turned a somatic cell malignant—a major step forward. Barry Marshall and Robin Warren were the first to demonstrate that bacteria, as well as viruses, could be carcinogenic—thus widening the focus of the inquiry. Finally, when Palmer Beasley discovered that hepatitis B caused liver cancer, it followed that the vaccine against it, which he tested extensively on the island of Taiwan, was also the world's first anti-cancer vaccine. We know that of the people alive today, about 2 billion have been infected with hepatitis B at some time in their lives. But now we also know how to reduce the grip of this lethal disease. As time goes by, fewer and fewer will have to struggle against it and its deadly effects—a story that most tumor virologists confidently expect will be repeated with other cancers as well.

Cancer is a burdensome disease. Worldwide, it costs $286 billion a year according to a 2009 report.[20] The disease touches almost everyone. Every year 12.5 million people will be diagnosed with it and 7.5 million will die. One in three people will develop it at some time in their lifetime; the other two will know someone who has it. In the middle of my work on the manuscript for this book, my husband, Gordon Cornwall, was diagnosed with melanoma. I know, firsthand, the lurch in the stomach that a diagnosis of cancer can bring and the ricocheting emotions that follow—fear, anxiety, confusion. And then while I was finishing the last revisions of the book in August 2012, I was saddened to learn that Palmer Beasley had suddenly died of pancreatic cancer. I remembered how vigorous he'd seemed when I interviewed him in December 2010, and I found it hard to absorb the news. With millions of others I share the hope that our familiar scourge will soon be conquered. A few scientists who noticed something slightly out of the ordinary and were curious about it have brought us closer to that day.

2

PALMER BEASLEY DISCOVERS A SILENT EPIDEMIC

I have not had the difficulty some scientists have had—getting outside the box.

—R. Palmer Beasley

THIS IS A DISASTER

On the evening of December 15, 1978, Jimmy Carter faced television cameras and quietly explained that the United States was shifting its international policy. Sitting at a plain wooden desk, in front of a gold curtain and flanked by two flags, President Carter said,

> Good evening. I would like to read a joint communiqué which is being simultaneously issued in Peking at this very moment by the leaders of the People's Republic of China: Joint Communiqué on the Establishment of Diplomatic Relations between the United States of America and the People's Republic of China, January 1, 1979. The United States of America and the People's Republic of China have agreed to recognize each other and to establish diplomatic relations as of January 1, 1979.

Shortly afterward, eight thousand miles away from Washington, the announcement crackled out over loudspeakers in the Navy base in Taipei, Taiwan. It was Saturday morning on the island, and Palmer Beasley

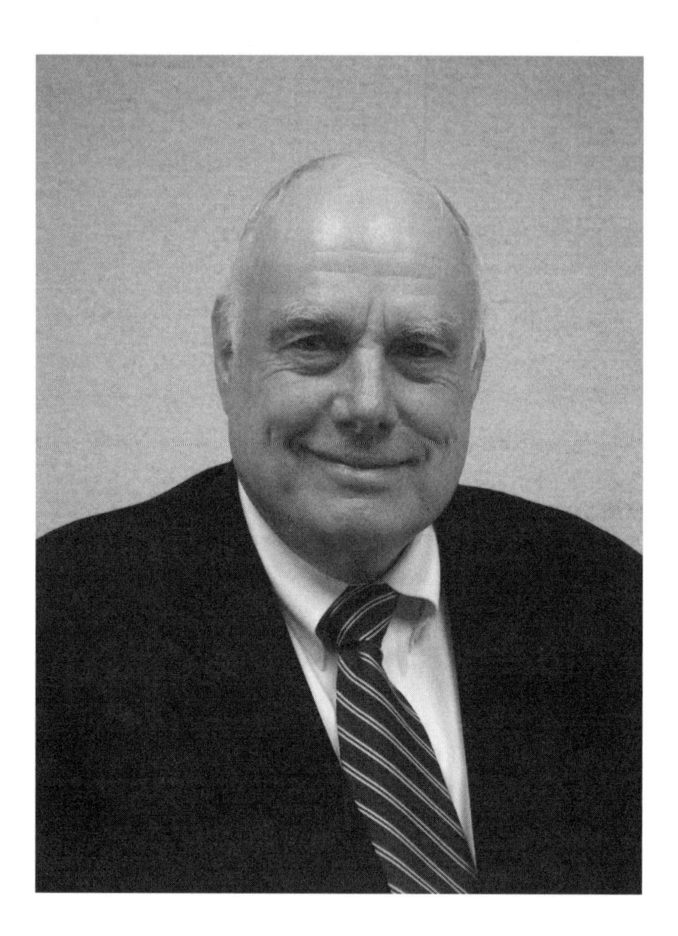

Figure 2.1. Palmer Beasley. Photo courtesy of University of Texas, Public Health Department

was in the PX, the base store, buying a few things in preparation for a Christmas trip back to the US. The news caught the forty-two-year-old doctor completely by surprise. He was stunned. "This is a disaster," he thought. "We're right in the middle of all this great stuff and suddenly there's the whole unraveling of relations between the US and Taiwan. All of our wonderful logistics and people are going to be pulled out from under us. We will no longer have a place to work."

Beasley was the head of clinical investigations at the US Naval Medical Research Unit in Taipei, usually known as NAMRU-2. Established in 1955, it was one of several research facilities the Navy operated around the world. This one was in a sprawling complex owned by National Taiwan University. It included both a hospital and laboratories where investigators had been chasing some of east Asia's most common microbes and viruses—cholera, trachoma, smallpox, rubella. Beasley was also an assistant professor of epidemiology at the University of Washington in Seattle. His department, which had established relationships with the local university and the Navy research unit, often sent faculty to Taiwan for several years at a time to investigate infectious diseases. But now the US was recognizing the People's Republic of China and severing its diplomatic ties with Taiwan. The Navy was pulling out—and the lab, of course, would be going too.

Beasley had moved to Taipei in 1972 to study hepatitis B. An inflammation of the liver caused by a virus, it was a bewilderingly complicated disease that affected people in multiple ways. It caused a range of symptoms: fatigue, joint pain, nausea, fever, headaches, and, at times, jaundice and severe abdominal pain. Some individuals recovered fully after an acute episode; others developed a chronic infection which often led to life-threatening liver problems. And some, while remaining healthy themselves, became carriers who transmitted the virus to others. Taiwan turned out to be an ideal place for Beasley's research. Though he didn't know it when he arrived, the island was one of the world's "hotspots" for hepatitis B.

By 1978, Beasley was close to making an important breakthrough. He had just begun a new trial which he thought would demonstrate how a vaccine could prevent babies from becoming carriers. He had also stumbled upon some provocative evidence that chronic hepatitis B was an important cause of liver cancer. He'd come across the data while he was helping a couple of University of Washington colleagues with a study they had set up in Taiwan of something quite unrelated—cardiovascular disease. The evidence Beasley uncovered was so suggestive that he got a grant from the National Cancer Institute to investigate the hypothesis that hepatitis B was a cause of liver cancer. During the past two and a half years, he had recruited thousands of Taiwanese civil servants to participate in a trial. They were a good representative sample of the island's male population—office workers, policemen, school teachers, university professors, customs officials. And conveniently for Beasley, they received a routine medical exam every couple of years as part of a health benefits package—something on which he could piggyback his own research. Beasley had just completed the enrollment of

23,000 apparently healthy individuals in his study. He had tested them for hepatitis B and was planning to follow their health status for the next twenty years, using reports from their medical exams and hospital records. If the study confirmed his suspicions, it would be a startling and significant finding.

Jimmy Carter had tried to be nuanced. Although the US was shutting its embassy in Taiwan and establishing another in Beijing, Carter assured his listeners that it would still maintain cultural, commercial, and other unofficial links with the people of Taiwan. He observed that the people of mainland China comprised one quarter of the Earth's people. The country was already playing an important role on the world's stage, and in the years to come, that was likely to grow. The US, he said, was just recognizing a geopolitical reality. Carter's address was short, only eight and a half minutes long. His manner was undramatic, understated even; nevertheless, for the people of Taiwan and the Americans who were working there, the speech was a bombshell.

Chiang Ching-kuo, the president of Taiwan, informed about Carter's announcement at 2:30 in the morning, said the move was "a great setback to human freedom and democratic institutions." He placed his army (500,000 men strong) on full alert, because he feared an attack from Mainland China. To avoid any political disturbances, he postponed the parliamentary elections which were scheduled to take place on December 23. Many ordinary Taiwanese were upset and confused by what had happened, as this news story shows:

> More than 2,000 demonstrators enraged by the normalization of US Chinese relations besieged the US Embassy and an American military compound. . . . The demonstrators . . . began hurling eggs and stones at the embassy, breaking some windows. From there the protestors marched to US Ambassador Leonard Unger's residence and on to the military compound. . . . At the compound they put up a poster declaring "Down with the US and Communist China." Some burned an American flag and raised the red, blue, and white flag of Nationalist China. A group of demonstrators then barged through the gate and a handful of Marine guards drove them back with tear gas.[1]

I'M NOT LEAVING

I met Palmer Beasley and his wife, Lu-Yu Hwang, a physician and his collaborator, in Seattle on a mild, moist Saturday in December 2010. The two researchers had come to visit family for Christmas and generously offered to sandwich in an interview. I had driven down from North Vancouver and we talked over lunch at Ray's Boathouse, an iconic Seattle seafood restaurant overlooking Puget Sound. As we spoke we could see boats, small and large, plowing through the waters outside the window.

Beasley was a tall, vigorous man in his mid-seventies—a dean emeritus of the school of public health at the University of Texas in Houston. He had given up his administrative duties, he said, and so was able to do what he liked best—epidemiology. I quickly discovered that he also liked to tell stories. I settled in to what I had a feeling would be an interesting interview.

I asked how it was that the Navy came to be interested in hepatitis B. Beasley said, "It was always asking, 'How can we help troop readiness?' That was their mission. They were interested in hepatitis B because they knew it was a problem in relation to transfusions, and certainly military people get transfusions." NAMRU-2 employed about 450 people and was essentially a three-way collaboration among the University of Washington, the US Navy, and National Taiwan University. Beasley recalled,

> It was an odd and sometimes uncomfortable fit. I was not in the Navy; I was a civilian working for a US university at a Navy facility that was housed in a building belonging to a Chinese university. I had some problems with the Navy but I also had a lot of help from them. They provided space and the space included high-level Chinese technicians and nurses assigned to me, paid by the Navy. I had a substantial team—twenty people for my projects. In addition, I was responsible for other laboratories and field epidemiology. I did some work for Tom Grayston [the first dean in the School of Public Health at the University of Washington], who was very interested in glaucoma. I also helped other people with some respiratory projects.

Beasley said that he personally found it easy to get along with most of his Chinese colleagues. Medical professionals usually spoke English, and many had studied in the United States. The US had maintained diplomatic ties with Taiwan ever since Chiang Kai-shek fled to the island in 1949 after losing the civil war with the Chinese Communists. Diplomatic relations between the two countries were not always easy. (Harry Truman once called Chiang Kai-shek a "usurper" and a "dictator.") But the people of Taiwan tended to have a warm regard for Americans, and Beasley's collaborators often became good friends. Charlie Lin was a professor of public health at National Taiwan University who had a knack for and an interest in computers, then a nascent technology. In 1976, Beasley bought one of the first personal computers in Taiwan, a Wang 22, but he had no idea that he needed programs to make it work. Charlie volunteered to help and figured out how to write software that would store and analyze data. "Charlie was a constant colleague," Beasley said. "He was unbelievably helpful. In 1975, my first wife left; she didn't like Taiwan and didn't want to stay. We had an unhappy divorce. Charlie provided support; he invited me to his home every day to have a meal at his house. We had an extraordinary friendship." There was George Lee, whom he had met at the University of Washington and whose specialty, pediatrics, made him a valuable resource. There was Chen Kung-pei, a distinguished professor of public health at National Taiwan University. Many people considered him to be the father of public health in the country. He'd died earlier in the year, but he'd been a great supporter and facilitator. And, of course, Lu-Yu Hwang, who just recently joined his research team as a postgraduate fellow, and who was quickly becoming a good friend too.

Carter's speech took most Americans in Taiwan by complete surprise, according to Beasley:

> People nearly fell on the floor. It was a terrible blow for everyone who was there. That meant that the US, including the Navy, was going to withdraw. For military people it was like, "Jesus, I wonder where we are going to go." Taiwan had a lot of US military at that point. There was an airbase, warships, a US Navy hospital, NAMRU-2. Getting everyone out was a big logistical undertaking.

After the announcement, the US Ambassador Leonard Unger advised all foreigners to keep off the streets. Palmer Beasley didn't believe that individual Americans would be in any serious peril even though relations between the US and Taiwan had changed at the highest levels. So scientist that he was, he decided to test the waters. "I remember saying to Lu-Yu, 'I'm going to go out into the street. I don't believe the people of Taiwan are going to endanger me.' She and I walked around a crowded downtown part of the city called Shi Men Ding. It was pretty much a normal sunny Saturday afternoon. I was completely right. The US Embassy people were utterly foolish."

Beasley decided there was no reason for him to go—and every reason to stay. He had no idea how the University of Washington would react to the changed political situation. But he was resolved to remain in Taiwan even if he had to leave the university in order to do so. He was deeply committed to finishing his research and answering important scientific questions about hepatitis B. On Monday, December 18, despite the turmoil, Beasley called a staff meeting. He said, "I didn't know anything about this. It was as much a shock for me as it was for you. I don't know what's going to happen to NAMRU-2. I'm not part of the Navy. I don't know any of that. But I'm not leaving." He told the group that, as he had already planned, he was going to California to be with his parents for Christmas. But, he said, "I'm coming back. We're going to stay and finish the project."

Beasley soon learned that even though the Navy was leaving, there was no rush for him to vacate the space he was using. But there were many other things Beasley didn't know. He didn't know if he would be able to keep the equipment he was using in his research. He didn't know how he would pay for the staff or services that the Navy had been providing. He didn't know for sure that the people who'd been working with him would want to continue to do so—although he was fairly sure they would. And he didn't realize that when the US Navy moved out, he would be left exposed to people in Taiwan who were suspicious of what he was doing—men like Dr. Wang Chin-mao. He was the sixty-five-year-old director of the Department of Health in Taiwan, a powerful official. Though he was a physician who had received a PhD in public health from Columbia University in New York, he was deeply distrustful of the idea of immunizing newborns. He thought it was risky and that if anything went wrong, he would be blamed. He didn't want any blemishes on his spotless record and would try everything he could to stop Beasley's research program.

On Tuesday, December 19, surrounded by a cloud of uncertainties, Beasley left to visit his parents in Los Angeles.

SNAKES AND LIZARDS

The tan Chevy station wagon slowly crept down the deserted road. It was 1948, and twelve-year-old Palmer Beasley and his nine-year-old brother, Bruce, were sitting on the hood, holding on to the hood ornament to keep themselves from sliding off. Their father, Robert, was driving. It was night, and they were travelling under a dome of stars. The Mojave Desert was surprisingly cool, though the road still held some of the day's punishing heat. The two boys kept watching what the headlight beams were illuminating.

"There," said Palmer, pointing. A red racer, the fastest snake in the desert. It could move at speeds up to seven miles per hour. Palmer and Bruce prized it above all because it was uncommon and difficult to catch. The boys slapped the hood of the car. Their father braked, and the two youngsters jumped off, moving quickly and surreptitiously toward the unsuspecting reptile. Palmer picked it up carefully and brought it back to the car. This was a mean-tempered snake, and though it was not poisonous, its bite could tear the flesh.

I spoke to Bruce Beasley on the phone at his home in Oakland, California. Now an internationally recognized sculptor, he remembered those trips into the desert vividly:

> Palmer got interested in animals, particularly snakes and reptiles. Dad was more than willing to go out on endless herpetology-oriented trips to the Mojave Desert and we spent many, many weekends camping in the desert, going out at night. That was the best way to collect snakes and lizards, because they would hide from the heat during the day. They came out at night. The desert would cool off a surprising amount, but then the roads would hold the heat. The warm roads at night were a wonderful place to catch snakes and lizards. People wouldn't let you do that now. Appropriately the animals are protected. But there were a lot of them then and the desert was not full of people riding motorcycles and four-wheel dune buggies. So we had a pretty serious animal collection. That was driven by Palmer. As the younger brother I was excited to go along with him.

At one time, the Beasleys' suburban home housed twenty-five snakes, including a boa constrictor, as well as an owl and a red-tailed hawk. This was a significant (and scientifically oriented) operation. The boys raised rats to feed the snakes and built cages in their backyard and basement. When the animals died, they dissected them and made skeletons, fastening their bones together and assembling them into full-scale models.

Palmer was born in 1936—a third-generation Angelino. His grandfather, Oscar, originally from Kentucky, had moved to Los Angeles around 1912. His father, Robert, was born there, went to Hollywood High School, and was in the first graduating class at the University of California, Los Angeles. Both men were bankers. Palmer, one of two boys, grew up in west Los Angeles, where he attended public schools. His mother, Bernice, was a public lecturer. The profession doesn't really exist anymore, but it has a history in the United States stretching back to the mid-nineteenth century. Bernice was hired to give talks on a variety of subjects—literature, psychology, and contemporary interpretations of society.

Palmer Beasley had no desire to follow in his father's or grandfather's footsteps. When I spoke to Bruce, he said, "It was clear from the beginning that Palmer was going to be involved in science of some kind." In seventh grade, Beasley began participating in a youth program at the Los Angeles County Natural History Museum which took youngsters on trips to introduce them to the local flora and fauna. He developed an enthusiasm for collecting animals, a passion which his father happily encouraged.

Beasley liked to go exploring and hiking. He was a Boy Scout and then an Eagle Scout, the highest rank it is possible to attain in the organization. Bruce recalled how broad his brother's interest in nature was. "I remember that he would wake me up at night and we'd climb up on the roof with binoculars and star charts and plot the heavens and learn about all of the different galaxies." One of Palmer's projects, a ninth-grade presentation, particularly impressed Bruce:

> Palmer had created the skeletons of four different animals by boiling them and taking the skeletons apart. He didn't create a three-dimensional model, but a flat, scientific layout of the bones. He carefully, carefully made a prominent list of the missing bones. You couldn't have got me to emphasize what was not there. I would have wanted to draw attention to what was there. Palmer explained to me that listing what was not there was just as important as listing what was there. I learned that intellectually, but emotionally I never really believed that. He recognized the importance of scientific truth as

opposed to a great presentation and drama. I, on the other hand, was more interested in the visual drama.

By the time he was in high school, Beasley was sure he wanted to be a doctor. "I was attracted to medicine. I knew and understood fairly early that it was a field with enormous breadth that allowed a lot of different choices." When he was eighteen he went to Dartmouth College, a small liberal arts school in New Hampshire. He said, "I was fascinated by the array of learning opportunities. I took way more courses than we probably were supposed to." He also managed to squeeze in being a scoutmaster in the nearby town of Hanover. Bruce said, "I think it's telling that as a student in a difficult program he ran thc scout troop for town kids. This wasn't a college activity. This was something he sought out on his own. That shows Palmer's sense of giving to the larger society."

At Dartmouth, Beasley enrolled in a full pre-medical course load *and* majored in philosophy. He remembered, "By the time I graduated, none of my humanities friends had any idea that I was taking premed. My medical friends had no idea I was doing humanities. I knew that philosophy was no way to make a living but I took it as an intellectual challenge." Beasley was "enchanted" with the Enlightenment, particularly by Hume and his discussion of causation. "Scientists have a tendency to get down into details. Collectively, they have the problem that they don't see the big picture, but philosophy is the big picture. I have not had the difficulty some scientists have had—getting outside the box. Philosophy is very helpful from the standpoint of thinking in different ways."

Beasley entered Harvard Medical School in 1962. Rather quickly, he decided that infectious diseases would be his focus. He was influenced by his exposure to people like John Enders, a professor at Harvard who received the Nobel Prize in 1954 for developing a way of culturing polio viruses. Beasley said, "I was very interested in finding an organism and a disease that were not understood. I picked hepatitis. At that point, it looked like the last, or at least, a major disease for which the cause wasn't known." The disease was old, reported for centuries. The Greek physician Hippocrates described an infectious jaundice in the fifth century BC, and many epidemics occurred in the nineteenth and twentieth centuries. A famous outbreak occurred in 1885 in Bremen, Germany, when two hundred shipyard workers who were immunized against smallpox subsequently developed jaundice. This was the first well-documented case of a vaccination-transmitted hepatitis infection. In the 1940s, a British doctor, F. O. MacCallum, made some headway in understanding the disease. He distinguished between two forms: infectious hepatitis, now called hepatitis A, which was passed on by contaminated water and food; and serum hepatitis, today known as hepatitis B, which seemed to be transmitted mainly by exposure to contaminated blood or needles. Palmer wanted to investigate hepatitis B. At the time, nothing was known about its connection with liver cancer; nevertheless, it was already recognized as the more lethal of the two diseases.

Scientists suspected that the agents causing hepatitis were viruses, not bacteria, because they could pass through fine filters. However, they were unable to grow them in the lab, which made it difficult to study them and their effects. By the mid-1960s, hepatitis research reached a discouraging deadlock. Beasley remembered, "Many people told me, 'Don't bother, it's not doable.' I said, 'I'm a young man—I need a big problem. This is just about the right size for me.'"

Beasley graduated from Harvard in 1962 and did an internship at King County Hospital in Seattle. He said, "I fell in love with Seattle in 1955 when I drove my roommate, who came from Seattle, home for a summer holiday. I thought this was the most splendid city I had ever seen. That got me wanting to come here."

SHOE-LEATHER EPIDEMIOLOGY

As we were talking about how Palmer's interest in hepatitis B began almost fifty years ago, he suddenly asked, "Does EIS mean anything to you?"

"No," I said.

"It stands for Epidemic Intelligence Service and was part of the CDC [the Centers for Disease Control, a cornerstone of public health in the United States]. It actually began in the mid-fifties. When I went there, it was early in its creation. It had from twenty-five to fifty young, mostly men at that time, brought in and trained to do the fieldwork for epidemics. So the investigation of epidemics, the core of people who did that was called the EIS." Known as officers, the young doctors who worked for the organization were dispatched to ferret out viral or bacterial culprits in communities all over the United States and even abroad—when other countries requested the agency's help. You could think of it as a medical CIA.

Like members of the Army, Navy, or Coast Guard, the EIS officers wore uniforms. In 1963, when Beasley joined up, doing so was a way of fulfilling National Service Requirements. Completing a tour for public health meant that Palmer wouldn't be drafted. "It doesn't seem reasonable that you could have so much fun and have it count towards your military service," Palmer said, shaking his head. I thought he was still a little amazed at his good fortune.[2]

Alex Langmuir, the director for twenty years, was passionate about a style of investigation known as "shoe-leather epidemiology." Academic epidemiologists often do their work far away from the events that gave rise to them by examining medical records and poring over documents. Langmuir had a different idea about how to do things:

> He emphasized the personal acquisition of raw data in the field: conducting face-to-face interviews, tracing the suspect food back to its origin, collecting specimens for laboratory analysis, pounding the pavement. Indeed, Langmuir so imbued the first EIS class with the shoe-leather approach that it is believed that they designed (in circumstances that now are beyond memory) a wry symbol for the EIS: the print of a shoe with a hole in the sole, worn through by persistent field investigations. This logo remains the proud emblem of the EIS.[3]

Physicians who joined the elite corps took a month of intense training, but Langmuir insisted that this was just an introduction to the subject. The real learning would happen out in the field—by doing. Beasley recalled, "It opened my eyes to a kind of epidemiology that was barely taught in schools and which municipal and state governments are usually not able to support. There aren't enough epidemics in cities to have a core of people dedicated to them. It does make sense to have experts collected on a national level; they can go and work where the outbreaks occur."

In the United States, Beasley looked mostly into "mundane" outbreaks—small occurrences of gastroenteritis or meningitis. But in 1965, he investigated an outbreak of *Salmonella typhimurium* that affected eighteen thousand individuals in Riverside, California. When he arrived on the scene, he didn't know how the disease was spreading, but he interviewed people who were sick and determined that the bacteria was in the water system. It was the largest outbreak of salmonella ever to occur in the United States.[4] Beasley also went to the South Pacific when a rotavirus caused a large gastroenteritis outbreak there. Young children often develop this infection, which results in diarrhea. It is a leading cause of death among children in developing countries.

Beasley flew to Bolivia twice to investigate bubonic plague. I was surprised by this; I thought plague was something we hadn't seen since the Middle Ages. But Beasley told me that a plague pandemic had occurred as recently as the late nineteenth century. In 1894, it spread rapidly from Canton and Hong Kong, carried by flea-infested rats on ships. Within ten years, it entered seventy-seven ports on five continents. Nothing so devastating has happened since, but Beasley recounted that there have been sporadic outbreaks—such as one in 1964 in Bolivia. The Pan American Health Organization informed EIS director Langmuir about it. He obligingly sent Beasley and another officer, Jim Gale, down to research the situation (and bring back a sample of the bacterium). The two Americans flew to La Paz and then penetrated deep into the Bolivian countryside, on horseback, by burro, and on foot. They found a Quechua settlement where thirteen out of the thirty-two inhabitants had caught the plague. At the time, antibiotics could successfully treat the infection, but the natives were so far from medical help that eight of those who contracted the disease died. Mindful of the duty to return with a bacterium, Beasley and Gale disinterred one of the victims. Gale donned a pair of gloves and cut off the finger of her right hand. He knew that the pathogen would survive better in bone marrow than anywhere else.[5]

Beasley recalled, "It was not only a very exciting way to spend two years, it also opened my eyes by allowing me to see a lot—how things were done in different states, different countries." Later he would do some of his most creative work in Taiwan with the assistance of doctors, nurses, and patients who were Chinese, and whose experiences and beliefs about medicine were often quite different from his own. His stint in the EIS was invaluable.

A NOVEL HYPOTHESIS

"Quite often when people do research," Beasley said, "they jump into it. By virtue of the fact that I couldn't jump in immediately, it caused me to think and plan more than others often do. It was evident to me that amongst the many things not known about hepatitis, the means of transmission was not known."

In 1965, Beasley returned to Seattle to do a residency in internal medicine and then a postgraduate fellowship in preventive medicine at the University of Washington. While there, he became convinced that the story commonly told about the spread of hepatitis B was incomplete. He said, "There was no doubt that a dirty needle would do it. It was also known that some people had bad blood and it could be transmitted during a transfusion." But he was struck by the evidence that this was not a new disease. "There wasn't enough blood transfusion, particularly in the past, to explain how the virus got around so well. There had to be another way in which it was transmitted." What might that be? Beasley asked his colleagues and mentors what they thought. "I got various answers like, 'Well, that's a really interesting question. Maybe sword fighting.' I laughed and said, 'You know, I don't honestly think there was all that much sword fighting most of the time. So, what else?'"

Beasley recalled, "I asked myself, 'What is the commonest way in nature, that people have contact with each other's blood?' The answer to that is very straightforward: mothers and babies. Every baby has a mother and therefore human contact with blood in that sense is very common. I thought, 'Before I look at anything else I think I should look at that.' That was the premise and the logic that went into exploring that hypothesis—that mothers were passing the virus to their babies, somewhere in the birth process." Beasley termed this a "shrewd guess."

The idea that a mother could infect her baby during pregnancy was not new. In 1941, Sir Norman McAlister Gregg, an Australian ophthalmologist, discovered that pregnant women with rubella could transmit the virus to their infants, who were then at risk for cataracts, deafness, and heart defects. At first, his finding was regarded with suspicion. In March 1944, an editorial about Gregg in the prestigious British medical journal *Lancet* stated, "He cannot yet be said to have proved his case." The piece went on, "The lay public have always held that congenital malformations have an extrinsic explanation—from being frightened by a dog to falling downstairs—and it will be strange if the influence of a mild illness in the first months of pregnancy, accompanied by a rash, has escaped attention."[6] In the 1940s, the problems Gregg attributed to a rubella infection were regarded as genetic in origin. It took him about ten years to convince the medical establishment otherwise.

You might think that this example would have helped Beasley to make *his* case. But rubella and hepatitis B are very different. Newborns affected by a mother's rubella infection usually have symptoms at birth. Hepatitis B, on the other hand, does not reveal itself until much later in life; the connection to something occurring during gestation is not obvious. When I phoned Timothy Block, a professor of microbiology and immunology at Drexel University College of Medicine and the president of the American Hepatitis B Foundation, to ask about the novelty of Beasley's hypothesis, he had this to say: "There are many examples of viral diseases that are transferred vertically. But when you're looking at those that are transmitted vertically *and* silently, well, hepatitis B was the first to be recognized." It took time, though.

John Fox, one of Beasley's professors, was clearly doubtful. When Beasley told him what he was thinking, Fox asked, "What gave you that idea?" Beasley remembered, "Nobody took me seriously. That was part of the theme all the way along. All the way through, people were highly skeptical. I now know that is characteristic of most new discoveries. People tend to be very conservative and therefore react in a negative way, sometimes a hostile way. In this case, at that particular time, [they were reacting] in a sort of bemused way. They thought what I was doing was admirable but my conclusion was funny." Despite the lack of enthusiasm from his instructors, Beasley began devising a plan for testing his ideas about what is called "vertical transmission." He knew that he lacked an important component of such an experiment—a tool for detecting the hepatitis B virus. Nevertheless, he prepared, to be ready for the day when such an indicator was discovered. His confidence was well placed. A marker soon became available, thanks to Dr. Baruch Blumberg, an inquiring American scientist.

Harvey Alter, who is now the chief of clinical studies in the Department of Transfusion Medicine at the US National Institutes of Health (NIH), was one of Blumberg's early collaborators. He spoke to me on the phone from his office in Bethesda, Maryland, and remembers Blumberg, who died in April 2011, "as a great thinker, who had very eclectic interests." He said, "He also was a great hypothesizer. He used to have a chart in his office that was almost a full wall. It was a list of his hypotheses. He would write down a hypothesis and then trace, with arrows, the experiment that should be set up, and the outcome of the experiments. Very often these hypotheses failed, but he never gave up. A failed hypothesis was just the beginning of a new hypothesis. He was inquisitive and had great perseverance."

Blumberg wrote a book about his work called *Hepatitis B: The Hunt for a Killer Virus*, but initially he was not looking for a virus at all. He was interested in polymorphisms, genetic variations that provide a selective advantage. In his book, Blumberg gives what he calls a "famous" example of one. Hemoglobin is a protein in the blood essential for the transport of oxygen. Most of us have a double dose of normal hemoglobin, HbA, because we inherit normal genes from both our mothers and fathers. However, in some regions of the world, a mutation of the gene which produces hemoglobin is common. Individuals who inherit two copies of the mutation produce a double dose of a variant of hemoglobin called HbS. They will develop sickle-cell anemia. On the other hand, those people who have just one copy of the mutated gene do not develop sickle-cell anemia, but are less likely to die from malaria. This explains the persistence of HbS in parts of Africa where malaria is endemic.[7]

Hoping to explain why some people are resistant to certain diseases (and susceptible to others), Blumberg wanted to discover more such inherited variations in the blood. He reasoned that hemophiliacs who received multiple transfusions probably encountered blood proteins that were different enough from their own to trigger the formation of antibodies. He could use their immune system as an exquisitely sensitive detector. Antibodies in the serum (the liquid component of blood) from hemophiliac patients would hone in on unusual proteins. Blumberg began collaborating with Harvey Alter when he was at the NIH Blood Bank. Alter was interested in why some patients developed chills and fevers after blood transfusions. He wondered whether they were suffering from immune reactions to the blood they received.

The two scientists used a technique called agar gel diffusion, which showed when an antibody from one person's serum found a matching antigen in another person's blood. The equipment was very simple; it cost less than $100 and involved a glass plate coated with agar gel. If there was an interaction between two sera placed on the plate, a telltale arc appeared. Alter and Blumberg began exposing the sera of people who had received multiple transfusions to the sera from healthy individuals in diverse populations. In 1963, the researchers ran one experiment in which they exposed the blood serum from a hemophiliac patient in New York to a panel of sera from twenty-four people. The serum from the hemophiliac reacted, all right—but with just one of the sera in the panel, that from an Australian aborigine. This showed that the hemophiliac had the antibody to something in the aborigine's blood. What could these two people from completely different parts of the globe have in common? The experiment also showed that the antigen, whatever it was, was rare, since the test only detected it in the serum of one individual in the panel.

Alter said, "We weren't looking for the cause of anything. We were looking for polymorphisms, and so what the experiment suggested was, 'Here is another serum polymorphism.' That it would have the impact it eventually had, didn't occur to us. I was a hematologist. Blumberg was a geneticist. Neither one of us had any background in hepatitis. It just shows you how undirected research can lead to big discoveries—not because you're looking for something, but because you find something and you figure out what it means."

Blumberg's curiosity was aroused. What had he found? Blumberg called the mystery substance "the Australia antigen" after the country of its origin. To learn more about it, he began looking for it in sera from all over the world. He found that the antigen was very uncommon among normal healthy people in the United States, but much more frequent among individuals in Africa, the Pacific, and Asia. It was especially prevalent in Taiwan. In 1965, Blumberg and Alter published a paper indicating that 13 percent of the population of Taiwan had it.[8] Then Blumberg discovered that leukemia patients were likelier to have the antigen than healthy people. This made him think he might have found a polymorphism which explained susceptibility to leukemia, and he started testing people with Down's syndrome, who are at a higher risk for this cancer. He found that they were more likely to have the antigen than other people. And then, said Alter, "he did a very clever study. He went further and looked at individuals with Down's in different settings—in institutions, lodges, at home, at birth. While the rate was very high in those who were institutionalized, it wasn't present at birth and it wasn't present in kids who lived with their parents. This was the first clue that it had something to do with the environment and the bad hygienic conditions in institutions—that it might be related to an infectious agent." In early 1966, Blumberg found one boy with Down's syndrome who was negative for the antigen at first, and a few months later positive for it. When he became positive, lab tests showed that he had developed chronic hepatitis B. This was the first indication that there was a link between the Australia antigen and hepatitis B. "The real clincher," said Alter, " was a technician in Blumberg's lab, Barbara Warner, who was working on this and was the control, the antigen-negative control in the lab. One day she was feeling terrible, tired and sick to her stomach. She was at work, so she tested her own blood. Lo and behold she was antigen positive. She had a classic case of hepatitis with jaundice. This was the clincher that this was related to hepatitis."

Blumberg began to test the hypothesis that hepatitis and the antigen were associated. By mid-1967, Blumberg knew that the frequency of the antigen was significantly elevated in people with acute hepatitis. Then he found that it was higher among patients with chronic hepatitis. Being able to detect this antigen started to have practical applications. University of Tokyo's Kazuo Okochi showed blood that tested positive for the antigen was much more likely to transmit hepatitis to transfused patients than blood that tested negative.[9] A study at the Philadelphia General Hospital indicated that when blood containing the antigen was not used in transfusions, the incidence of post-transfusion hepatitis B dropped by two-thirds.[10] By the end of 1970, Blumberg knew he had not detected a polymorphism at all. He had identified an antigen on the surface of the hepatitis B virus (HBsAg). The surface antigen was not in itself infectious, but it indicated the presence of an infection. In 1976, Blumberg was awarded the Nobel Prize for his remarkable discovery.

At the time, there were 150,000 cases of post-transfusion hepatitis every year in the United States.[11] But if Beasley's intuition was right, most people around the world who acquired the disease did not get it from a blood transfusion, but from their mothers. Post-transfusion hepatitis was just the tip of the iceberg. There was a vast and largely hidden epidemic yet to be discovered. However, before Beasley could map its contours, one more development was necessary. He needed to be in a place where he could see the iceberg. That happened early in 1969 when a rubella (German measles) outbreak occurred in Taiwan, just as a newly created vaccine against the disease was ready to be tested. Tom Grayston, Beasley's mentor, had established connections with National Taiwan University and NAMRU-2. As well as sending young faculty from his school to the Navy facility on two- to three-year tours to conduct research, Grayston had also done some studies himself in Taiwan. He could mount another one quickly and left for the island to determine the epidemiology of the rubella outbreak and the effectiveness of the new vaccine. He took some of his postgraduate fellows along with him to help with the field investigation. "This," said Beasley, "is what got me to Taiwan."

The epidemic lasted about two years. Beasley shuttled between Seattle and Taipei, spending several months at a time at NAMRU-2, directing teams of scientists and organizing a laboratory. While he was getting his name in the rubella world, he was also pursuing his own interests on the side. He read everything he could about hepatitis and began developing a network of local contacts. Taiwan was a poor country that was not technologically advanced. Few people drove cars, for instance. However, the working conditions were good. The standards of education and training for medical people were high, and many were eager to collaborate with American investigators. Beasley introduced himself to Dr. Julia Tsuei, the chief of pediatrics and obstetrics at the Taipei Veterans General Hospital, a large teaching hospital. She was interested in his ideas and receptive to the possibility of working together.

The more time Beasley spent in Taiwan the more it grew on him. It was a vibrant place, its markets bustling, brimming with fresh fruit and vegetables as well as locally caught seafood. There were many blossoming trees, cherry and plum, and an abundance of flowers—chrysanthemums, rhododendrons, lilies, orchids, and roses. Beasley said, "Most people don't realize that the highest mountains in Asia outside the Himalayas are in Taiwan. They have snow-capped mountains that look like that," he said, pointing to the peaks we could see beyond Puget Sound outside the window. "Good for hiking?" I asked. "Absolutely," he said.

By 1972, Beasley was an associate professor at the University of Washington. His work on rubella was finished, and Grayston gave him the opportunity he coveted—an assignment to NAMRU-2 to study hepatitis B. He went with a pediatrician, Cladd Stevens, who was completing her master's degree in public health at the University of Washington. Beasley said, "It was all coming together. I had my tool. And by this time, having had the idea of mother-to-infant transmission, I had actually designed a protocol to study it in Taiwan. I was able to start more quickly than anybody else that I know of who went to a foreign country. I knew what I was going to do and who I was going to do it with. My timing couldn't have been better."

A WONDERFUL RESULT

When Beasley got to NAMRU-2, a Navy scientist, Dr. Karl Anderson, had already started a small study at the Taipei Veterans General Hospital about the transmission of hepatitis B from mothers to babies. "We were able to build on that," recalled Cladd Stevens when I spoke to her on the phone. The Taipei hospital was both a veterans' hospital and a general hospital with a busy maternity ward. Families were large in those days; women often had four, five, six children and there were many pregnant ladies. The hospital was well organized with high levels of prenatal care and follow-up. It was an excellent place to do research. Beasley went to see Julia Tsui and explained that he wanted to confirm his idea that hepatitis B was transmitted vertically. She thought it was a reasonable hypothesis and gave him her permission to go ahead.

Beasley's idea was to test women who were coming to the maternity ward for prenatal care. When their babies were born, he would test them right away and then at regular intervals thereafter—one month, three months, six months, a year. He was planning to use a new assay that improved on the sensitivity of Baruch Blumberg's test, so that he could detect even the mildest of infections being passed from mothers to their babies. As he prepared to get consent from the patients, some of his Chinese colleagues warned him that his plan would never work. No mother would want him to take blood from her baby. He could try, they said, they had no objections, but they were sure none of the mothers would agree. When Beasley said he thought they would agree, his colleagues told him that he just didn't understand the Chinese. They hated to give blood, and they really didn't like the idea of bleeding a baby. They would just say no.

Beasley went ahead anyway and asked the mothers if they would like to participate in his study. He told them what he was trying to do and why it was important. He said he didn't have a vaccine for hepatitis B yet, although his goal was to get one. He pointed out that the risks for the baby were minimal although he would be sticking a needle into their arms. He also explained that they could withdraw from the study at any time. Beasley said,

> We learned that the Chinese mothers were very concerned about their babies' health and about contributing to something bad for the baby. They knew that hepatitis was very common and they knew it was bad. We also learned that Chinese mothers were often very afraid of their mothers-in-law. A common story was that a woman would agree to participate, come back, sometimes in tears, and say, "I want to do this but my mother-in-law won't let me." We told her to explain what we were trying to do. She'd say, "Oh, she won't listen." We'd give the mother a description of the project in English and Chinese. We'd also give her our telephone number and tell her that we were happy to talk to anyone. They liked that. Sometimes the husbands would come in and sometimes the mothers-in-law. The fact that we were open about it, not hiding or resistant, that appealed to everybody.
>
> Sometimes it was that the mothers-in-law thought taking blood from the baby would hurt it. I would say there was probably a complexity of feelings and thoughts, but in part, it was just related to the amount of education. Less-well-educated people would be more resistant. The young men and women that had a high school education generally understood that a body replaces blood, that taking blood is a medical procedure that's accepted, and there wasn't a lot of anxiety about that.

Cladd Stevens remembered that they tried to make it as easy as possible for the women to take part. Instead of asking them to come back to the hospital, a team followed the babies entirely through home visits. "We also provided well-baby advice," said Beasley. "The Chinese clinics tended to be very busy and with very little communication between the doctors and the patient. We gave the mothers a lot of time, so they really liked that. It turned out that we got most people to agree. As these studies evolved, a high proportion of the babies born in Taipei were participants."

The results of Beasley's first trial were remarkable. Within a couple of months, Beasley found that 15 percent of the women he was testing were positive for hepatitis B, even though they showed no signs of it and seemed perfectly healthy. Very few of them had a history of recent blood transfusions, injections, or acupuncture. By the time the babies of infected mothers were three months old, 40 percent of them were positive too.[12] Like their mothers, they seemed perfectly healthy. Beasley told me, "The babies looked just fine—happy and normal." But he began to suspect that these early infections were related to Taiwan's high rates of chronic liver disease.

Most of the babies who eventually tested positive began to do so around the time they were three months old. If the incubation period for babies was the same as for older children and adults—about ninety days after exposure—this suggested that they became infected during the birth process. Beasley explained, "We thought then, and we still think, that the placenta is squeezed during the trauma of birth. This causes some tiny little tears in the placenta and little bits of blood get squeezed across the placental barrier from the mother into the baby. Up to that time, the placental barrier, the membrane that separates the mother from the baby, is intact and prevents the virus from going across." Only a few of the babies, less than 5 percent, were positive at birth. Beasley believed that they had probably been infected earlier—at some time during the pregnancy.

"It was a wonderful result," said Palmer Beasley, beaming across the table at me. To him it meant that intervention might be possible—at least for those babies who didn't acquire the virus while in the uterus. When I asked Beasley whom he first told about his discoveries, he said that he and Cladd Stevens discussed them and then talked to Dr. Julia Tsui and Dr. I-Sen Shiao, who worked under her and was in charge of pediatrics. They were "positive, enthusiastic, interested, and happy to facilitate further study." Beasley also informed people at the University of Washington. "John Fox's reaction was, 'Are you sure?' This was entirely appropriate. After all, it was such a new finding that more work had to be done to confirm it," said Beasley. The results were published in the *New England Journal of Medicine* in March 1975.[13]

This was a major breakthrough, but there was much more to learn about hepatitis B. Beasley kept on studying the disease, trying to develop a complete description of it. He found that breast-feeding did not seem to have any effect on transmission and also that babies born by C-section were at the same risk as those who weren't. He travelled all over Taiwan, taking blood samples even in remote communities. He said, "I had worked with Native Americans, Alaskan natives, on a number of different projects. I'd worked in South America. I was pretty prepared to deal with people. I knew instinctively that the way to deal with them is with respect and honesty." His ability to think on his feet also helped.

> We asked the local school if it was okay for us to do this [collect blood samples from the children] and the school was okay with it. Then we sent home notes to the families asking permission. The teachers said, "We don't think the families will agree," but a high percentage did.
>
> I remember one seventeen-year-old girl. We lost track of her paperwork. We bled her without the form. It was an oversight. We always intended to have signed consent. The father came over and he was furious. The girl said, "It's okay, Daddy." She was fine with what had happened. Her father, though, was jumping up and down mad. He said, "You are going to take the blood to Taipei, send it to the US, and sell it." I thought to myself, "This is a terrible accusation. How am I going to counter it?" I called my nurse over. I asked her to get the biggest syringe she had, and to have several more in readiness. Then I asked her to bleed me and when she was done, hand me the syringe. I took it and squirted the blood on the ground. I wanted to show the father that we had plenty of blood and we didn't have any need to sell it. His jaw dropped. By the second one, he was convinced. It was a totally effective demonstration.

It soon became clear that the Chinese, whether they lived in Asia or other parts of the world, were particularly subject to hepatitis B. Their carrier rates were higher, and Chinese mothers were more likely than others to pass on the virus to their children. Naturally, this led some people (Baruch Blumberg among them) to speculate that the Chinese had a genetic disposition to the disease. But Beasley was able to show that this was not the case. When he was studying the vertical transmission of hepatitis B, he learned that the fathers of the babies had a rate of infection similar to the mothers—about 15 percent. But their carrier status did not seem to have much influence on whether the babies became infected. If the disease were genetic, then they would have a discernible impact.[14]

While the surface antigen showed that an individual was infected with hepatitis B, another antigen indicated whether a person was likely to pass on the virus. Lars Magnius, a Swedish researcher, discovered what he called the E-antigen. Beasley said, "We were able to show that those mothers who were not E-antigen positive did not transmit to their babies and virtually every E-antigen–positive mother did. This was enormously significant. Then we were able to show that in other populations around the world, it was the E-antigen rate that varied in different ethnic groups." Beasley added, "It's still not clear why these E-antigen rates are different. Some people think it's due to the genetics of the people; others think it's due to the genetics of the virus." In any case, discovering the E-antigen was useful. Beasley could predict with almost 100 percent accuracy which infected mothers would pass the virus on to their children, and where intervention would be most needed.

Once someone was infected, what determined whether that individual developed a chronic form of hepatitis B? Age turned out to be the critical factor. Beasley did a series of careful studies to illuminate this issue. He found that about 95 percent of babies infected at birth became carriers, whereas less than 5 percent of people who were infected at eighteen did so.[15] This suggested that as people matured, their immune systems became more capable, and they were better able to throw off the disease. The vast majority of adults did not need any medical intervention to fend off the virus. Newborns were another story. If infected, very few of them were able to repel the virus on their own. A vaccine for neonates was one solution, but creating one was uncharted territory. Newborns were known to respond poorly to most vaccines—which is why infants usually receive immunizations some months or weeks after birth.[16]

TOO IMPORTANT TO LET GO

Hepatitis B affected three out of every twenty people in Taiwan; most of them got the disease from their mothers at birth. There were other modes of transmission—unprotected sex, dirty needles, contaminated razors. But when the virus travelled these "horizontal" pathways, it encountered individuals whose immune systems were generally more robust, and it wasn't able to take root—to colonize the potential host so successfully. In Taiwan, hepatitis B was nourished by vertical transmission.

Beasley knew that to combat the epidemic, he had to intervene at birth. He thought, "If the mothers are transmitting, I'm going to give immune globulin to the babies, to try to prevent the disease." Also called gamma globulin, this blood product provided virus-fighting antibodies. It was known as passive immunity (and contrasted to active immunity). The individuals receiving the ready-made protection didn't acquire the appropriate "memories" to replenish the supply, as they would if they had active immunity. Passive immunity was just short-term, but it was a way of buying time. If the gamma globulin neutralized the hepatitis B virus when the babies were most vulnerable, their immune systems might be able to develop an active response later.

Beasley had contacts with Cutter Laboratories in Berkeley, California, because he had used their immune globulin in his rubella studies. He said, "Cutter saw the potential immediately," and it offered to send him some. Beasley said, "Everybody liked the idea. Immune globulin has a good safety record. And having established that the babies were getting something bad, giving them something to prevent them from getting it had real appeal. We had no problem getting collaboration. Julia [Tsui] was very happy to participate; the families were happy to take part." He set up a randomized, double-blind study with three arms—comparing a placebo, standard immune globulin, and hepatitis B—specific immune globulin (derived from the blood of donors who had particularly high levels of antibodies to hepatitis B). He sought participation from mothers who were E-antigen positive and were thus, without intervention, almost certain to infect their children.

For Beasley there was one great unknown about this study. How long after birth should the globulin be given? The only examples described in the medical literature were trials with "needle stickees"—usually medical personnel who were accidentally jabbed with hepatitis B—contaminated needles. In those investigations, the immune globulin had been given within seven days of the incidents, so Beasley decided to do the same for the babies in his study. He had them injected with immune globulin within a week of being born. Unfortunately, the results were not impressive. By twelve months, babies who received the globulin were just as likely to be carriers as those who got the placebo.

Nevertheless, in March 1978, Beasley flew to San Francisco to present his findings at the Second Annual Symposium on Viral Hepatitis. The weekend of March 17 was warmer than usual; the city basked under sunshine and azure skies. Despite the weather, Beasley felt depressed. He would have liked to be presenting a more positive outcome. There was only one small glimmer of hope in the data. As it turned out, not all the babies received their shots within the same time period. Those born on Friday afternoon waited the longest for their globulin and those born on Monday morning had the shortest wait. Only one group seemed to have benefited at all from the procedure—those who had received the injection within forty-eight hours of being born.[17] But since the general result was not encouraging, Beasley didn't see how he could convince anyone to fund another study using this approach.

One of the people in the audience at the symposium was Dr. Saul Krugman, a professor of pediatrics at New York University, a widely known expert on multiple infectious diseases—chicken pox, measles, hepatitis. He was sitting in the front row—his usual spot in conferences and presentations. When Beasley was finished, he leapt up and said, "Palmer, you must repeat the study and you've got to do all the injections immediately after birth. I will see that you get the money, this is too important to let go." Beasley remembered, "When I mentioned that I was worried because the results weren't as good as I was hoping for, Krugman shook his head, 'No no, you've got wonderful results,' he insisted. 'They just have to be expanded and confirmed.'" Krugman was as good as his word. Beasley got the money he needed from the National Institutes of Health and the US Food and Drug Administration. He began to plan for a second trial.

Back in Taiwan, Beasley got a call from a young woman, Lu-Yu Hwang, who had just completed her residency in pediatrics at the National Taiwan University Hospital. She had written a paper about infectious meningitis that she wanted to publish. She had translated it into English, but a professor of hers, Dr. Xu Chen-ging, had suggested that she ask his friend, Dr. Palmer Beasley, to check the English. Beasley had a reputation for avoiding editing tasks like this, but for some reason, he made an exception for Hwang, perhaps because Xu was his friend. He agreed to meet, and after he had looked at Hwang's paper, they went for lunch in the NAMRU-2 cafeteria. He told her about his research and said he was looking for a postgraduate fellow to work on the second phase of the immune globulin trial. He thought someone with a background in pediatrics would be well suited and wondered if she might be interested. Lu-Yu was intrigued, and although she was making plans to study in the United States, she decided to postpone them for a year in order to join Beasley at NAMRU-2.

Just around the time Hwang joined Beasley's research team, Beasley began to face numerous hurdles. The first occurred when Julia Tsui, who had supported and encouraged him, left the Veterans Hospital and moved to Hawaii. Without Tsui at the helm, the atmosphere in the maternity ward was no longer so congenial. Beasley faced criticism from one of the doctors who thought that getting an infection early in life was good. This was true of some diseases—adults are much more likely to suffer paralysis as a result of polio than infants, for instance. But the evidence was accumulating that this was not the case for hepatitis B, that an early infection caused serious problems later in life. Beasley couldn't seem to convince his colleagues of this, however. He decided to change institutions and made arrangements to run the second globulin trial at two other hospitals in Taipei—The Maternity and Child Health Centre and Mackay Memorial Hospital, run by a Presbyterian Mission.

THE CANCER PART SEEPED IN

When I asked Beasley how he discovered the link between hepatitis B and liver cancer, he said that it was quite different from his discovery of vertical transmission. He had come to Taiwan with the intention of testing his hypothesis about vertical transmission. But he had no suspicion that hepatitis B had any connection with liver cancer. He said, "The idea of vertical transmission was cerebral." He figured it out; it was a solution to a puzzle. "The cancer part seeped in. A number of pieces of the story came to impress me—that these were closely related." It began as part of his effort to do a thorough epidemiology of hepatitis B. He was interested in knowing who was getting infected and at what ages and how it might be related to other diseases. He thought it was striking that almost all liver cancer patients were hepatitis B positive. In addition, many people who didn't drink alcohol suffered from cirrhosis of the liver—a permanent damage or scarring which inhibits normal metabolic functions. Seventy percent of cirrhosis victims were positive for hepatitis B. Beasley said, "Everybody told me they didn't know what caused liver cancer and didn't know what caused the cirrhosis in the people who didn't drink." He thought to himself that there was a heavy burden of liver disease associated with hepatitis B in Taiwan. "The conventional way that Americans looked at this information was to say that people with liver disease were more susceptible to hepatitis B infection, but that the virus had nothing to do with causing the cancer. But it didn't strike me that way. It was a point of instinct, rather than a firm conclusion."

At the time, many oncologists believed that liver cancer was caused by aflatoxins. These are poisonous compounds found in moldy food—particularly cereals, oil seeds, spices, and nuts. Aflatoxins had been found in Africa and linked to liver cancer there. But Beasley couldn't find them in Taiwan where the food was fresh and abundant. There wasn't any malnutrition that might lead some people to eat lower-quality food. Although aflatoxins might explain liver cancer in Africa, Beasley didn't think they were relevant in Taiwan. There had to be another account. What was it?

The clue lay in research that ostensibly had nothing to do with liver cancer or hepatitis B. As soon as Beasley arrived in Taiwan, he began helping a couple of colleagues at the University of Washington, Dr. Robert Bruce and Dr. Russ Alexander, who had set up several studies of cardiovascular disease in Taiwan. Wanting to know whether the Chinese diet protected people from it, they had started a small cohort study involving about 3,500 men. They had collected blood samples to look for blood lipids—mostly fatty acids and cholesterol. Every year, the participants had an annual checkup, and Beasley was responsible for storing and tracking all the data. The real revelation came when Bruce asked whether there had been any deaths from cardiovascular disease. "There weren't any, no myocardial infarction [heart attacks] or strokes," Beasley said. But there had been deaths, and Beasley decided to find out what caused them. The first answer was "cancer." No information about the type of cancer was given, so Beasley asked the hospitals if he could send some of his assistants out to look at the chart records of these patients. It turned out that most of them were dying of liver cancer. When he looked at the blood samples that were stored on these patients, he found that they all were positive for hepatitis B and—

remarkably—that they'd had it before they developed liver cancer. "I was knocked out. I was just, 'Oh, my goodness!'" Then Beasley got one more piece of information. Over the past ten years, when people died in Taiwan, the government had collected data on the cause and the age and sex of the person. But no one had ever run this data through a computer and compiled it. Beasley arranged to do that—hired a truck, picked up a decade's worth of data cards from the local hospitals, and analyzed them. He found that among cancers, liver cancer was the third-highest cause of death in men, and the seventh cause of death among women. Beasley said, "It was all fitting together, the high carrier rate, the vertical transmission, and the high rates of death from cancer. Then I put together a grant application."

Beasley got funding from the National Cancer Institute (NCI) to investigate the relationship between hepatitis B and liver cancer. In late 1974, he began to recruit participants. It was remarkable that he received money for a study like this, since it ran counter to a popular theory of the day—that chemicals were to blame for cancer. The NCI officer assigned to the project thought it was remarkable too—but not in a good way. When he came to visit Beasley in Taiwan to discuss the research he said, "We want you to change the focus and study the lifetime food history of the Taiwanese."

This meant that the officer wanted him to look for aflatoxins in the local diet. Beasley was not enthusiastic, in part because he had already looked at this without any fruitful outcome. He said, "How much additional money will you give me?"

"No, no, I want you to change the project," said the officer.

"George," Beasley replied, "I have a specific hypothesis that I was funded to study. If NCI wants me to look at aflatoxins, I will work with NCI to develop a protocol to do it, but I will need additional money."

"You're not serious about this. You're not really suggesting that hepatitis B causes liver cancer, are you?"

"George, that's what I am suggesting," Dr. Beasley said.

"Don't be ridiculous, Palmer," the officer retorted. "If you said that in Bethesda you'd be laughed out of the place."

"I'm sure he thought I was difficult, problematic," Beasley told me, laughing. But there wasn't anything the officer could do. The grant had been approved, and since no more money was forthcoming, Beasley proceeded with what he had planned already. Almost 23,000 apparently healthy government employees agreed to take part in his study. He tested them for hepatitis B markers—the famous hepatitis B antigen as well as hepatitis B antibodies. Then Beasley began tracking their health status, using the results of yearly medical checkups, as well as hospital records. When any of the men died, Beasley took advantage of insurance reports which listed the cause of death. If liver disease was implicated, he recorded the information. The project was comprehensive, and Beasley was pretty sure it would verify what he had already seen with the small cohort study that had sent him down this path. But he needed time to accumulate, collate, and tabulate the data.

I COULD PUT YOU IN JAIL

It was January 1979. Carter's announcement had come and gone. Beasley had come back from his Christmas holiday in California and found that the US Navy was busily making preparations to leave. Beasley was committed to staying in Taiwan, but without the Navy which had provided much supporting infrastructure it was more difficult to carry on. Beasley told Captain Kurt Sorensen, the commanding officer at NAMRU-2, that he wanted a donation of the lab equipment and other machinery. Beasley said, "He was completely unwilling to say anything other than 'I don't know, maybe. Don't count on it.' This was in complete contrast to the folks at the US Navy Hospital who told us they would be happy to coordinate transfers of equipment."

So there Beasley was in a cavernous four-story building, watching as the Navy stripped it of everything it had brought and installed. Beasley told me that he remembered seeing the air conditioners sitting in crates ready to be shipped to Manila, NAMRU-2's new home. And how, shortly before they were scheduled to be loaded on trucks and taken away, Kurt Sorensen gave the word. Beasley could have them. Then the telephone company arrived to shut down service to the building. Beasley rushed over to the phone company headquarters with Lu-Yu Hwang and pleaded with a representative not to cut them off. The phone company employee said he would transfer the system to Beasley, who would then assume legal responsibility for it. Beasley filled out the appropriate paperwork, and when he thought he was done, the official asked him, "Where's the chop?"

"What chop?" Dr. Beasley asked, perplexed.

"The US Navy chop," the representative said. "The *original* NAMRU-2 chop."

Chinese chops are an ancient institution. Originally made of stone, they dated back to a time when many people were illiterate. They bore a carving of the name of an individual, family, or business and were dipped into ink in order to stamp documents or letters. The seals could be passed from generation to generation. If a father closed a business deal and signed a contract using the family seal, but died soon after, the son could carry on with the contract if he had his father's chop in hand. The chop was proof of the transfer of authority. That's why the phone company was so insistent on seeing the original stamp. Prints made from it didn't have sufficient gravitas. They weren't proof that Beasley was now in charge.

Beasley was dismayed. He thought to himself that Americans probably wouldn't keep a chop. They wouldn't appreciate its significance. He went back to the NAMRU-2 building with Hwang, worried and perplexed. How was he going to deal with this? His feelings must have been obvious because when he got back to the office, his Chinese bookkeeper, Josephine Shu, asked him, "What's the matter, Dr. Beasley?"

"We've got to have the original chop," he said, "but I'm sure the Navy didn't keep it."

'Dr. Beasley," Shu said," I know where it is."

"What?" said Beasley, astonished.

"It's in the back of a desk in the administration office. None of the Americans know what it is, but I know what it is."

Beasley hurried downstairs with Shu. He could see desks were being packed up. Maybe the one with the precious NAMRU-2 chop in it was already on a dock somewhere ready to be loaded on a ship. But Shu located the desk, pulled open a drawer, and said, "Dr. Beasley, I've got it!" Then he dashed back to the phone company.

"Good," said the official. "Now we can make the transfer."

Beasley recollected, "The first few months of 1979 were super-hectic—just with logistics."

And there was more trouble brewing. When the Navy pulled out in March 1979, Beasley's legal situation changed. The Navy had what is called a Status of Forces Agreement (SOFA) with the Taiwan government. This clarified the terms under which the US military was allowed to operate in a foreign country. American personnel working for the Navy were also covered by the agreement. It meant that the Navy took responsibility for what civilians like Beasley did while working in Taiwan. However, once the Navy pulled out, the onus for overseeing Beasley's activities fell directly to Taiwan. In particular, it fell upon the country's Department of Health, which Wang Chin-mao, a physician, had been directing since 1974.

Beasley had known for some time that Wang was suspicious of him. When the distinguished and eminent Chen Kung-pei died in February of 1978, Beasley had attended the funeral. Chen had made many contributions to the advancement of public health in Taiwan. Anyone who was anyone in the medical world in Taipei came, including, of course, Wang Chin-mao. Beasley recalled, "I tried to use that as a way to talk to Wang, but he wouldn't let me get close to him. He physically moved away. He wouldn't talk to me. He made it clear he didn't want to have any discussion."

Wang was worried that there would be some unfortunate result associated with Beasley's research, and that he would be blamed for it. He was especially concerned about what might happen if Beasley began to test a new vaccine that Merck Sharp and Dohme (today known simply as Merck) was in the process of developing in the United States. Beasley had already been testing gamma globulin to see whether this might prevent newborns from becoming carriers. But Wang saw gamma globulin and a vaccine in quite a different light. In the one, the newborn received antibodies; in the other, the baby got a shot of something derived from a virus. To Wang, this was inherently much riskier. "While to us it was a continuum," Beasley said, "to him it was very different."

In October of 1979, Beasley decided to see whether he could import the vaccine into Taiwan despite Wang's reservations. He was a little concerned about Merck. He thought that in view of the uneasy and uncertain political situation, the company might become reluctant to supply him with vaccine. To Beasley it seemed prudent to act sooner rather than later—to ask for the vaccine before the relations between Taiwan and the United States deteriorated any further. In order to bring in the vaccine, however, he had to apply for approval from Wang's administration. He knew that Wang himself would probably not approve, but he thought that perhaps if his application went through the normal channels, a lower-ranking official would see it as a routine matter, and rubber-stamp the document. Beasley was right; he was able to import the vaccine and, in fact, he was the first person in Asia to receive it.

Beasley began a series of immunogenicity studies to see whether the new vaccine actually stimulated the production of protective antibodies. He recruited mothers who were at low risk for transmitting the virus. And because he knew that newborns were especially vulnerable to hepatitis B, and he wasn't sure how they would respond to the vaccine, the first subjects he chose were older children. He said, "We took five- and six-year-olds, then two- and three-year-olds, then one-year-olds." The results were surprising. The younger the children were, the more their immune systems were stimulated. "It kept working so well," he recalled. He tested one group and got a good result, then tested a younger group and got an even better result. "It was wonderful. It was fabulous." The children and infants quickly produced substantial levels of antibodies without any adverse reactions.

The results were positive, yet puzzling. As the paper that Beasley and his colleagues wrote about this research states, "The question of why neonates handle HBV [hepatitis B virus] infections so poorly and yet respond so well to vaccination remains unanswered. We are unaware of analogous phenomena with other infectious diseases. Further understanding of the immune system at the beginning of life is needed."[18]

Whatever the reason for the babies' response, it was a stroke of luck. The next logical step was to start a trial with newborns whose mothers were at *high risk* of transmitting the virus. Ultimately, Beasley wanted to know whether he could help the babies who were likely to become infected. He was ready and eager to proceed with this, but events intervened. The popular press in Taiwan had serious questions about the immunogenicity studies. Were they safe? Why was Beasley "experimenting" on Chinese children? Why didn't he use American children? And why was the Department of Health so irresponsible as to allow a foreigner to expose local children to such risks?

Beasley responded by explaining that he was conducting vaccine trials in Taiwan rather than the United States because Taiwan had an epidemic of hepatitis B, but the United States did not. His explanation did little to allay fears. Wang Chin-mao sent for Beasley. He was taken to a tiny room with no windows. When Wang walked in, he wouldn't shake hands. Red-faced, he paced up and down in the cramped space.

"I could put you in jail," he yelled.

"For what?" asked Beasley.

"You imported the vaccine against the law."

"I imported the vaccine *with* the law."

"That's impossible."

"Dr. Wang, I did."

Wang sent one of his officials to investigate. After a few minutes, the bureaucrat returned with a piece of paper. "Dr. Beasley is right," he said, waving the stamped permit in front of Wang's face. Beasley was allowed to keep the vaccine. But further studies were out of the question for the moment. On March 17, 1980, a headline in one of the local newspapers, the *Central Daily*, stated, "The safety of Hepatitis B vaccine has not been proved, Department of Health disallows the trial on our children." A department of health official was quoted as saying, "Only if the American government permits the use of this vaccine in humans, will we let our children have the vaccination."[19]

Merck, the vaccine maker, began to hear stories about what was happening. Beasley said, "Overseas Chinese in the US told them that things were going to hell in Taiwan. They [Merck] called me and said, 'We hear it's all in the papers, you're really in trouble. You're about to be put in jail.' I said, 'It's okay. One thing I'm certain of is that I haven't done anything I'm ashamed of, or that is illegal.'"

IS CANCER A COMMUNICABLE DISEASE?

While the attacks in the newspapers continued, Beasley was getting results from other studies he had already launched. By June 1980, he was seeing his deep suspicions about liver cancer and hepatitis B borne out. When he looked at the health status of Taiwanese government employees, he found forty-nine cases of liver cancer among 3,454 carriers. On the other hand, among 19,253 non-carriers, only one developed the disease. The relative risk of primary liver cancer for carriers was many times that of non-carriers—273 times higher, to be exact.[20] You get a sense of just how risky hepatitis B is when you compare it to the hazards posed by smoking. For male smokers, the chance of developing lung cancer is twenty times higher than for nonsmokers. This makes lighting up dangerous to be sure, but not nearly as dangerous as hepatitis B. Beasley had discovered a cancer epidemic, passed on from generation to generation, inexorably and silently. Though it affected nearly 15 percent of the population, no one knew it was there. Beasley said that these results shocked everyone. "People wondered, 'How could the whole world have missed it? How could something that big have been sitting there?'"

Ludwik Gross, whom I mentioned earlier, and who discovered that female mice can pass on a leukemia-causing virus to their offspring, had considered the possibility of humans spreading a cancer-causing virus the same way. He thought that for several reasons, this disease-transmission from one generation to the next might occur unnoticed. While a captain in the US Army Medical Corps during World War II, Gross reflected about these issues in a paper called, "Is Cancer a Communicable Disease?" First he contrasted "vertical" transmission, an infection passing from a mother to her baby, to the more familiar type of contagion. He wrote: "In a normal or 'horizontal' epidemic, that of smallpox or common cold, for instance, the chain of infection spreads among individuals of the same generation and the whole picture of a communicable disease, as such, is clearly discernible to anyone; thus, several hundred consecutive cases of transmission of the disease from one individual to another may occur within a comparatively short time and certainly within the lifetime of the human observer." When it comes to vertical transmission, however, Gross noted, "one human observer can see but a very few scattered links in the chain of communication. The comparatively short life of the investigator does not permit him to follow the spread of the disease for more than a few consecutive transmissions, and the communicable nature of the disease may therefore entirely escape the individual observer." Gross pointed out that while a physician could visit a dozen victims of smallpox or the common cold in a day, to see a dozen victims of a vertical epidemic would require travel in the fourth dimension—time—as well as space. Gross also observed, "Another reason apparently responsible for the difficulty in understanding the problem of cancer is the fact that most of those who spread the disease are latent carriers; they do not themselves display any apparent symptoms, but many of them develop tumors upon reaching old age, or under the influence of certain hormonal or, as yet, obscure stimuli." At the time, no human cancers were known to behave this way. Yet Gross thought they might, "that human cancer may be similar to that observed in mice, and may also, perhaps, be communicable from one generation to another." It was a prescient essay; it took almost another forty years before anyone found what Gross surmised might exist, below the surface, out of sight.[21] I will have more to say about latent infection later in this book. My interview with Paul Ewald will explore why vertical infections are apt to be latent.

Because Beasley knew that hepatitis B had a primary role in causing liver cancer, he also knew that the vaccine trial he wanted to start was actually the world's first anti-cancer vaccine. Naturally he was anxious to begin; every delay meant that more babies would not be protected from a deadly disease.

In August 1980, the results of the second immune globulin trial rolled in. In this study, Beasley only looked at babies born to very high-risk mothers. He compared infants who received a placebo with those who got hepatitis B–specific immune globulin (HBIG). Some got one dose at birth, others got three doses (at birth, three months, and six months). Mostly the nurses injected the babies within minutes of being born. Beasley said, "Their instructions were to wash the baby and get the Apgar score [a rapid assessment of the baby's health]." If the baby was normal and healthy, they would give it HBIG. "It worked like gangbusters," Beasley recalled. "We hit it exactly right." Seventy-seven percent of the babies who received three doses did not become carriers. (This was better than those who received one dose—55 percent of those did not become carriers.) Among babies who got the placebo, only 9 percent did not become carriers.[22] Beasley said, "Everybody looked at our numbers and said, 'Wow.'" The data was unequivocal: gamma globulin could prevent even the most infectious of mothers from passing on the virus in a solid majority of cases.

Beasley learned something else from the study. HBIG is passive immunity, the transfer of ready-made antibodies from one person to another. Normally after a few months, it disappears. But, Beasley said, "We quickly saw that while some babies were protected and lost protection after a few months, other were passive-active. That was a new finding and a surprise. Passive-active was a known phenomenon, but nobody had seen it with infants or with hepatitis. It startled everybody." This suggested that HBIG contained some hepatitis B antigen which was stimulating the babies' immune systems to manufacture their own antibodies. It also suggested that HBIG and a vaccine could work in concert—that the presence of ready-made antibodies didn't prevent the immune system from making its own home-grown antibodies. Perhaps the combination would achieve even better results than what Beasley had seen so far. But to find out, he needed to run another trial. In the current climate, that was looking increasing unlikely.

I'M HERE TO MAKE A DECISION

The media coverage was relentless. So Beasley began waging a public relations campaign of his own:

> It's hard to be in the newspaper every day. You feel like hunkering down. But I thought this was the time to stand up and speak to as many people as possible. I spoke at the university. I told everybody I would tell every part of the story. I would answer every question. I said if there was information we didn't have, I would get it. That helped, and so did the fact that we had pristine science.

Beasley also knew that in the end, no matter how successful these talks were, it probably wouldn't change Wang's mind. "He was dead set against what I wanted to do," Beasley recalled. To get anything done, he had to go to the highest level—to the one person who had power over Wang—Premier Sun Yun-suan. Sun, who was sixty-five, had graduated from Harbin Polytechnic University in northeast China, majoring in electrical engineering. He had trained in the United States, working as an engineer on the Tennessee Valley Authority. In 1946, he moved to Taiwan to take a job with the Taiwan Power Company. He got the electrical grid up and running in five months after it had been destroyed during the war. From 1969 to May 1978, he had been the minister of economic affairs, whose goal was to bring sleepy agrarian Taiwan into the twentieth century. Beasley thought there was a good chance that Sun would be sympathetic to what he was trying to do. "But I couldn't just knock on his door—I needed an introduction." Beasley began planning how to climb the political ladder, introduction by introduction, step by deliberate step. He thought there was one man in Taiwan who could introduce him to Premier Sun—Li Kwoh-ting.

Li, sixty-nine, was a minister without portfolio, with access to everyone in the government. A physicist, he had studied at the University of Cambridge in England. His mentor, Lord Ernest Rutherford, discovered the concept of radioactive half-life (for which he had received the Nobel Prize in 1908). Li returned to China in 1937, then moved to Taiwan and entered public service there in 1953. He had been the minister of economic affairs and the minister of finance, before taking on his present role. Like Sun, his ambition was to modernize Taiwan. Beasley thought he would be interested in his research aims. But Beasley couldn't knock on his door either—he needed an introduction to him too.

It turned out that the way to Li was through a family friend of Beasley's, Beverley Brooks Floe, a well-connected American woman. She came to visit Taiwan in 1980, for a happy occasion. Palmer Beasley and Lu-Yu Hwang were getting married. While Floe was in Taiwan for the wedding celebrations, she introduced Beasley to a lifelong friend of her father's, Hu Kung-piao. Hu had met her father while they were both studying at the Massachusetts Institute of Technology, and they had kept in touch ever since. After Floe left Taiwan, Beasley thought that perhaps Hu might have an idea about how to approach Li. He paid him a call, and Hu did have a thought—Yen Chia-kan. A scientist by training, Yen had graduated with a degree in chemistry from St. John's College, a western-style university in Shanghai where English was the language of instruction. He'd held various posts in the Taiwan government, including minister of finance and premier (in 1963). When Chiang Kai-shek, the president of Taiwan, died in April of 1975, Yen assumed the remaining three years of his term.[23]

Hu introduced Beasley to Yen, who at the time was the chairman of the Council of Chinese Cultural Renaissance. At seventy-five, he was a dignified elder statesman, but his knowledge of Taiwan's political landscape ran deep. He quickly understood that Wang was an immovable obstacle and also appreciated the significance of Beasley's research. Yen promised to get him an interview with Li, and in due course, Beasley received a message that he would be picked up and taken to see the minister without portfolio. At the appointed hour, a black car arrived and Beasley got in, alone as requested. He told me he had the impression that if it didn't work out, Li wanted the evidence of their discussion to disappear. Beasley was taken to the headquarters of what was called

n imposing stone building on Zhongxiao East
; something like visiting the West Wing of the
ngton.
urage of people reporting to him, but in that first
e any phone calls or countenance any interrup-
complete attention. After he explained his busi-
important. How can I verify what you've said?"
ve him information and a list of names of people
who would vouch for him. Li said that they would
wo weeks. "I want you to prepare some visuals.
y that the busy premier can understand. I want to
ou present is very clear." He also told Beasley that
o put Taiwan on a solid financial footing and now
some money, he was looking for good ways to
ant people just buying fancy cars. His dream was
nce and technology juggernaut.

Beasley returned for another meeting, this time with graphics and pictures. Li liked what he saw. "Good, good, good," he said as the illustrations scrolled past. He arranged a brief informal meeting with Premier Sun and explained that a formal discussion would follow. At the formal meeting, in December 1980, Beasley was invited to bring some of his staff, so he took Lu-Yu Hwang. The premier had about twenty advisors. Most of them had a science background; among them were the president of National Taiwan University, the head of the National Science Council, and, of course, Wang Chin-mao. Beasley told the group that if Taiwan made a decision to permit a trial of the hepatitis B vaccine, it would have a chance to lead the world—to show everyone else how to deal with this serious epidemic. Then the premier led a question-and-answer session in English. Wang Chin-mao sat there looking red-faced and resistant. Beasley told me, "I don't remember if he was crossing his arms, but he might just as well have been. The premier then turned to him and said, 'It's pretty clear, we need to get ready to do a vaccine study. Dr. Wang, what do you say?'"

Dr. Wang sputtered. "We have to hold committee meetings."

The premier exploded. "God dammit, what are you doing? I'm here to make a decision. And I've made a decision. We're going to do this. You better get your committees together pretty quick." The premier gave him a date. "You have till February," he said.

Beasley recalled, "As I went out of that meeting, one of the participants told me, 'You sold your story perfectly. If I were Dr. Wang, I would turn in my resignation now. You just saw something that no foreigner ever sees.'"

Wang could not resist Sun. On February 19, 1981, the *Central Daily* had a positive story about the vaccine for a change. The headline read, "Staff of American Institute in Taiwan (AIT) Accept Hepatitis B Vaccine, Confident of This Still Experimental Vaccine." Beasley was interviewed for the story, and when asked why Americans were willing to take the experimental vaccine he explained, "First, they were afraid of getting hepatitis; second, they had solid confidence in this vaccination."[24] The next day: Wang's retreat. The *Central Daily*'s new headline read, "Hepatitis Vaccine Is Permitted," although Wang Chin-mao, who was interviewed in the article, was careful to point out, "Parents can withdraw their children from the experiment at any time after they decide to accept the vaccination."[25]

TURNING TO GOLD

In November 1981, Beasley finally began the vaccine trial. Merck was still worried about him even though he had Sun's support and Wang's permission. The pharmaceutical giant agreed to supply vaccines, but not to pay for anything else—salaries or other operations. Beasley said that Merck "misread how problematic it was and failed to stand behind us." Taiwan's National Science Council, the Far East Foundation, and the Yuan Chih Memorial Fund stepped in with more funding.

Again Beasley recruited mothers who were E-antigen positive and greatly at risk of transmitting the virus. The enrollment went quickly; despite all the negative publicity surrounding his work, Beasley found that many families were happy to participate. He gave 159 babies HBIG (hepatitis B-specific globulin) at birth and administered the vaccine to them at three different intervals. A group of 84 babies, who were the controls, received neither HBIG nor vaccine. By December 1982, all the babies were at least nine months old and Beasley could analyze what had happened. He found that 94 percent of the babies who received HBIG and vaccine did *not* become carriers. It was a significant improvement over either the vaccine or HBIG used alone.

On the other hand, 95 percent of the controls, who received nothing, were infected by the time they were three months old. It was a stunning difference.[26]

Timothy Block termed Beasley's discovery that it was possible to interrupt the transmission of hepatitis "remarkable." He said, "No one would have thought that you can give a vaccine and gamma globulin post-exposure and do any good. There's apparently a very small window of time after you are born. It should be too late, but for some reason it's not." He explained why it was so urgent to act at the time of birth: "Your immune system is going around and doing a taste test on every cell in your body. When it sees an antigen, it makes a memory and says, 'That's self. Never hurt, never attack that.' If hepatitis antigen is present in your body at that time, your immune system will declare it as 'self,' and it will be unable to make good antibodies against it." Once the hepatitis antigen is labeled "self," it is invisible to the immune system and settles in for the long haul, a chronic infection. For the intervention to succeed, it must occur before this happens. Block said, "If you are infected from your mother you have to interrupt transmission within twenty-four hours of birth, whether by vaccine or gamma globulin, preferably both." It's not much of an opportunity, but it is enough.

Beasley's troubles with the Taiwanese government were over. "We had turned to gold," he said. "Everybody was happy to cheer. The people who had stuck with us in the toughest times—Lu-Yu, George Lee, Charlie Lin, C. L. Chen—those people had courage. It was tough on me and I wasn't Chinese. But they were being slammed in their own country." Taiwan acted quickly on the knowledge that Beasley had acquired. In 1984 it adopted the world's first nationwide at-birth hepatitis B immunization program—the application of the world's first anti-cancer vaccine. Cladd Stevens explained, "Palmer was terrific. He convinced everybody that Taiwan could become a model for hepatitis B prevention for the world by taking the opportunity through long-term follow-up to show that preventing hepatitis B virus infection would also prevent liver cancer. Dr. D. S. Chen's paper published in the *New England Journal of Medicine* was the first to show that the population incidence of liver cancer declined following a nationwide hepatitis B vaccination program.[27] That was a terrific part of the story. It was the icing on the cake. That proved that it was preventable." Then Thailand followed Taiwan's example.

Beasley tried to convince the leaders of the World Health Organization (WHO) to incorporate HBV vaccine into its routine childhood immunization program. At first, they resisted the idea. They were reluctant to endorse an immunization program that would require immunizing babies at birth and they worried that it might compete with routine vaccination for diphtheria, polio, tuberculosis, and measles. Finally in 1992, after attending many meetings, Beasley succeeded. Immunization against hepatitis B became part of the WHO's global childhood vaccination program.

Liver cancer usually strikes adults, so it will take time before the full benefits of the HBV vaccine are realized. However, already it is achieving some positive results—fewer children are developing the malignancy. Dr. Chen's study showed that the rate of liver cancer in Taiwanese youngsters aged six to fourteen had halved between 1981 and 1994. More recently, in 2009, a study published in the Journal of the National Cancer Institute tracked two thousand children and teenagers aged six to nineteen in Taiwan and found that the rate of liver cancer was down by 70 percent since the introduction of the national vaccination program.[28]

Beasley's research highlighted the danger of viral liver disease and, following his lead, scientists have been working hard to identify additional hepatocellular pathogens. We now know that in addition to HBV, five other viruses attack the liver—hepatitis A, C, D, E, and G. Hepatitis B still affects the most people—350 million. Hepatitis C is second, at 170 million. Like hepatitis B, C also causes liver cancer, but unfortunately, so far there is no vaccine.

Beasley received numerous scientific awards. In 2011, the National Infectious Diseases Foundation gave him the Maxwell Finland Award for Scientific Achievement for his distinguished career in preventive medicine. Cladd Stevens, who was at the awards dinner, said,

> In his talk he made an interesting point. The question was whether it is possible to eradicate hepatitis B, as it has been possible to do with smallpox. There's a small amount, less than 10 percent of hepatitis B, that is transmitted from mother to baby in utero. These mothers have very high viral loads. He explained that to eradicate hepatitis B you have to eliminate the in-utero infections. Because the vaccine cannot prevent them, anti-viral therapy may be required. The thing that impressed me was that he had taken up this banner as well. He

was not giving up. He was motivated by a clear insight into really finishing the story. It illustrated his commitment to keep going until the problem was finally solved.

Dr. Beasley died in August 2012 of pancreatic cancer. The *New York Times* obituary stated, "Dr. Beasley had hoped to see hepatitis B eradicated in his lifetime. That goal was not achieved."[29] The banner must pass to someone else.

MILLIONS OF STORIES LIKE MINE

Even though Beasley did not see the eradication of hepatitis B, he achieved a great deal. Hepatitis B was a major epidemic. Globally, about 600,000 people still die every year from the disease and its associated illnesses—more than a person a minute. Hepatitis B is responsible for 80 percent of liver cancer cases, and 560,000 people who develop liver cancer from it die. Where hepatitis B is endemic, the economic burden is crushing. A 2009 study in *Value in Health*, a journal of the International Society for Pharmacoeconomics and Outcomes Research, reported that in China, alone, the costs of hepatitis B and its associated illnesses might be as high as $15 billion (US) a year.[30]

However, the vaccine is beginning to make inroads. Many lives have already been saved. According to the WHO, a billion doses of hepatitis B vaccine have been dispensed worldwide since 1982. In countries where 8–15 percent of children used to be chronically infected, the infection rate has plunged to less than 1 percent. By 2011, 179 countries were vaccinating their infants against hepatitis B.[31]

Another way to measure the scale of Beasley's accomplishment is to talk to people like Arline, a woman who was diagnosed with hepatitis B in 1988 at the age of thirty-nine. At the time she lived in Toronto, where she went through a battery of tests to determine why she felt so tired and nauseated. At first, they revealed nothing, and it looked as though her problems might even be psychosomatic in origin, not physical. Finally her doctor told her she had hepatitis B. She didn't have jaundice or an enlarged belly, other symptoms often associated with the illness. But a blood test was conclusive; the virus was active in her system. A doctor explained that she could hope for a remission, but the disease would probably stay with her for life. "No cure, no treatment." The words pulsed through Arline's mind like a drumbeat as she left his office.

Arline is now sixty-two. When she got her diagnosis, she was a working mother of three children. Speaking on the phone to me from Wilmington, Delaware, where she now lives, Arline told me that she was born in Shanghai and grew up in Hong Kong. At eighteen, she left for North America to seek higher education. She went to university in Wisconsin and, after graduating, married and moved to Toronto. She has a vivid memory of her struggles with hepatitis B:

> It works like a flip-flop. The virus will go to sleep and you won't be able to find it. But it will be reactivated once in a while. You never know when; it could be when your immune system is down. Then you feel lousy lousy lousy for four to six weeks. If you're young, you recover. You feel better and you forget about it. It's just as if you had a bad flu. A lot of people don't know they are infected. It is a silent killer. When the hep B is activated it's called a flare. You feel helpless and listless when you're in a flare. You are so bone-tired that all you can think is "let me sleep." I am very strong-willed and I forced myself up in the morning, Monday to Friday. I jumped in my monkey suit and went to work. Then I came home and collapsed. But I had three kids. I couldn't stay in bed all weekend long and not do anything. I had my first daughter when I was 25 so she was just a teenager. My youngest was very young. It was terrible.

Arline said that as soon as she was diagnosed, "public health descended. They wanted to test the whole family—my brothers and sisters, my mother, father, extended family. They documented it, who had it and who didn't." It turned out that of Arline's five siblings, four of them had hepatitis B. Her mother and all of her five siblings had it as well. Arline says, "There's no way all my uncles and aunts could have got it unless my grandmother was affected too. And she could very well have got it from *her* mother." Arline continued, "My uncle passed away a couple years ago. He was sixty-nine and he had primary liver cancer caused by hepatitis B. My cousin, my aunt's son, passed away with liver cancer at forty-nine. His sister was also affected." Arline's mother, an eighty-two-year-old resident of Toronto, developed liver cancer in January 2010. She was lucky; the tumor was small and it could be treated. Today, cancer-free, she goes out to play mah-jongg every day. Though she is beating the odds, for most people, liver cancer is so deadly they usually die within a year of the diagnosis.

"There are millions of stories like mine," Arline said. Families like hers have to deal not only with grief, but also with the economic fallout that occurs when productive members of the family are struck down in their prime. And in many parts of Asia, families have to cope with shame and stigma as well. Arline explained:

> In China, if you are a hepatitis B carrier, you have no life. You are the lowest of the low. You can't get a job, you can be discriminated against. Now the government has said you cannot be discriminated against, but they do discriminate—especially in rural areas. Shame and stigma is well ingrained in people's culture already. No matter what, if someone has hepatitis B he or she will not tell you about it. They are so afraid that if they tell somebody they have hepatitis B, nobody will socialize with them, nobody will invite them. Nobody will want to eat the food they prepare.

A proven treatment was not available when Arline first became sick. She participated in a few clinical trials of experimental drugs, some of which helped a little. Then in the late 1990s, she was part of the trial of a drug called Entecavir. It worked by interfering with the replication of the hepatitis B virus and made Arline feel much better than she had on the other drugs she had taken. In 2000, she moved to the US for career reasons, but stayed in the clinical trial and continued with Entecavir. Encouraged by Arline's response to the medication, her US doctors increased the dose and, she said, "that really put the virus to bed. They haven't been able to detect any virus activity in me for seven years now. It's a miracle drug. I would be six feet under without it." Still Arline suffers the consequences of having had the pathogen active in her body. She bruises easily, and her platelet count is low. (Platelets are cell fragments that provide the hormones and proteins necessary for blood clotting.) Arline said, "If I get a cut, I don't stop bleeding. In the winter, I cough up blood." Arline's liver is in such poor shape that since 2004, she has been on a list to receive a liver transplant. In 2006, she was forced into early retirement from her job with the bank ING Direct. She couldn't keep up the pace; the long hours her job demanded were too much.

When Arline got the hepatitis B diagnosis twenty-three years ago, her two daughters and her son were immediately tested as well. All three were positive, although the virus was dormant and they didn't have any symptoms. Arline said, "When you're young, you're strong. You can suppress the virus. But you never know. The virus may become active. This is the danger of hepatitis B." It also means that Arline's children are carriers. While they might experience no health problems of their own, they could still pass the virus on.

But the disease which had affected at least four generations of the family would not march on to a fifth. Arline's daughter, who lives in Toronto, has two youngsters, aged three and six. They were both immunized within hours of being born. This was followed by a couple of booster shots—a standard procedure recommended by the Canadian Public Health Agency. By nine months, the children had developed antibodies against hepatitis B; they were protected from the disease for life. Although Arline's children need annual checkups to monitor the virus, her grandchildren are completely free of it. Arline says, "They are not carriers, they don't need to be followed." Her family has suffered from a devastating scourge, but finally the cycle is broken. Her grandchildren are safe from hepatitis B and its fatal consequences—cirrhosis of the liver and liver cancer.

"We have the opportunity," said Arline, "of wiping this disease out in the next generation."

3

HARALD ZUR HAUSEN SOLVES THE RIDDLE OF CERVICAL CANCER

Let me say it this way. In order to succeed, we had to continue for a long time.

—Harald zur Hausen

KEY BISCAYNE, DECEMBER 1972

On a warm drizzly weekend in early December 1972, forty scientists crossed over a drawbridge to the island of Key Biscayne in Florida. Though within sight of Miami, the tropical getaway was like another world. The local Crandon Park Zoo boasted a pride of lions and in the mornings, golfers on the links could hear them roaring. The spot was a favorite of Nixon's. He met Kennedy there after losing the election in 1960—at Eisenhower's insistence. "Meet him or you'll look like a sorehead," Ike's wire read.

The weekend happened to coincide with the launch of the last American lunar mission. But the investigators converging on the luxurious Key Biscayne Hotel had a different achievement in mind—a medical breakthrough. They were elite, top-flight researchers from a variety of backgrounds—doctors, virologists, immunologists, biologists, pathologists. As they gathered around one large, doughnut-shaped table in the hotel, excitement was in the air, a feeling of being on the cusp of something big. The select conference was the brainchild of Dr. George

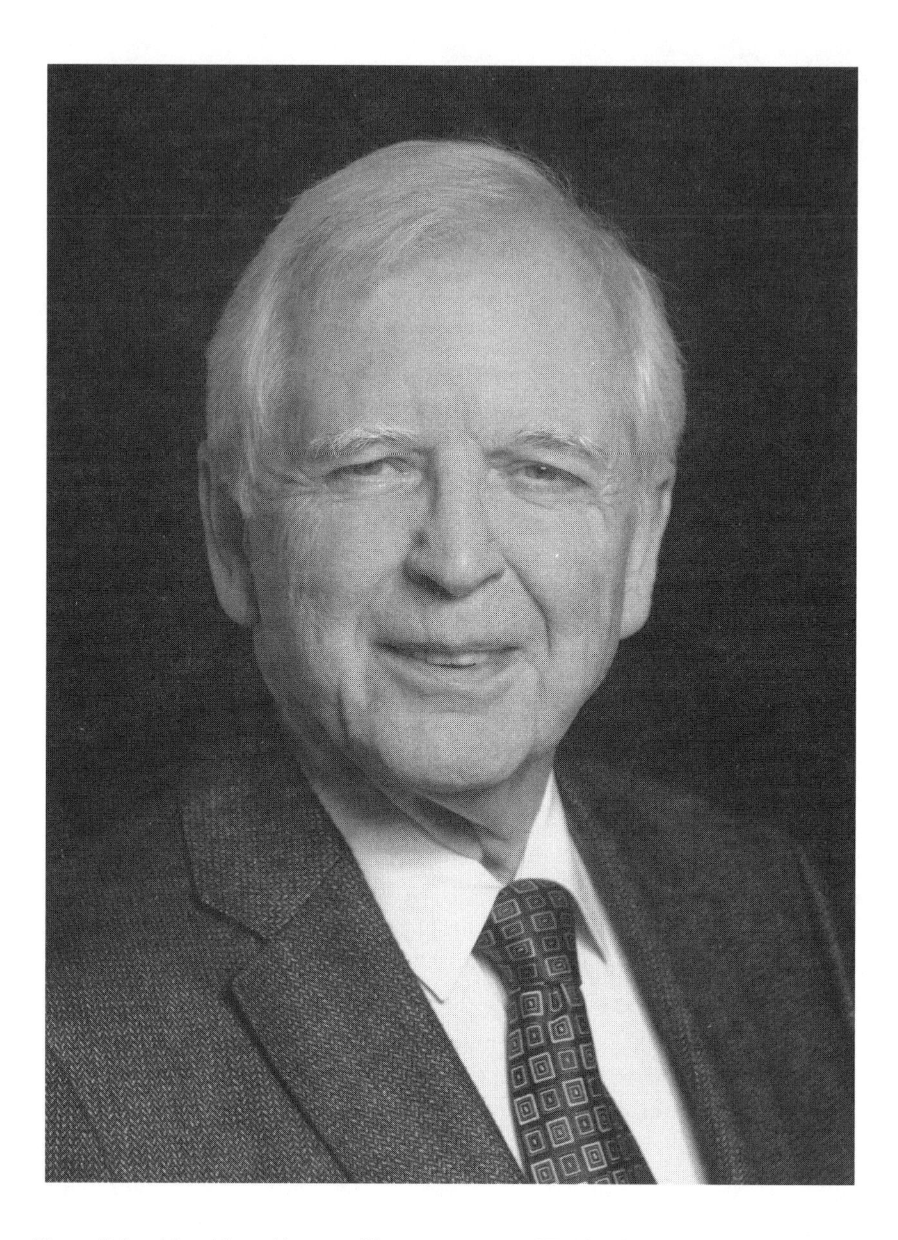

Figure 3.1. Harald zur Hausen. Photo courtsey of Tobias Schwerdt

Wilbanks and Dr. Clyde Goodheart from Rush Medical College in Chicago. They organized it because a significant advance seemed to be coming tantalizingly closer.

The topic was cervical cancer, a leading killer of women worldwide. The scientists at the Florida meeting were pretty sure that women caught the disease mostly from their sexual partners. Reports stretching back to the nineteenth century found that prostitutes were more likely to develop it than nuns, suggesting that a sexually transmitted disease spread the cancer. But which one was to blame? Syphilis, gonorrhea, and chlamydia were all potentially guilty. During the late sixties, however, a flood of research pointed to one culprit—a strain of herpes. "We virologists in the herpes field were riding a wave of popularity," Goodheart recalled, when I phoned him in his office. (He is now a cofounder and chief scientist at RexaDerm, a biotech company near Miami.)

The virus was an old enemy. The ancient Greeks knew about it and noticed the way distinctive sores inched over the surface of the skin. (Their word meaning "to creep" gave rise to the name "herpes.") The pathogen, which takes many forms, is responsible for diseases in both animals and people. Most of us are familiar with herpes simplex type 1, the cause of cold sores. Its close relative, herpes simplex type 2, results in painful lesions on the genitals.

By the sixties, the sexual revolution was in full swing, and the rate of genital herpes infection was rising rapidly. Stories in popular North American magazines and newspapers covered the phenomenon in lurid detail, ringing alarm bells about an epidemic incubating in colleges. Then a doctor at Baylor College of Medicine in Texas, William Rawls, published an influential paper showing that the infections might be more dangerous than anyone realized. He found that women suffering from cervical cancer were likelier to have antibodies toward genital herpes—indicating a previous infection—than were those who were cancer-free.[1] Suspicion about the virus was heightened when studies demonstrated that Epstein-Barr virus was implicated in a cancer that plagued children in equatorial Africa. It too was a kind of herpes. Although the malignancy, Burkitt's lymphoma, which attacks the immune system, was rare in Europe and North America, it helped to establish a general principle—herpes *could* be carcinogenic. That principle was further bolstered in 1970, when American farmers began deploying a vaccine that protected chickens from a highly contagious cancer, Marek's disease, also caused by a herpes virus. Prevention of the illness saved the US poultry industry millions of dollars and gave oncologists hope they might achieve an equally dramatic result with an anti-cancer vaccine for women.

In the way of most academic conferences, speaker after speaker discussed careful step-by-step progress on different fronts. As they presented mounting evidence implicating genital herpes, one man listened with growing uneasiness. He was Harald zur Hausen, a researcher from southern Germany, a rising star in scientific circles. Just thirty-six, he was already a professor and the chairman of the Virology Institute at the University of Erlangen-Nürnberg. Unlike most of the people at the conference, however, zur Hausen believed that genital herpes was the wrong suspect. It might be present at the scene of the crime, but it was not the perpetrator. He wanted to share his belief—and the negative data that supported it, even though, as he wrote later, "negative results have always had a lower priority than new discoveries." But he thought the emphasis was misguided. He observed, "It would be interesting to find out how many scientists have repeated the mistakes of others thereby."[2]

Viruses are tiny parasitic particles, about a hundred times smaller than most bacteria. Not much more than packets of genetic material in a layer or two of protein, they are unable to multiply by themselves. Instead, they commandeer the reproductive machinery of other organisms. The host cells end up duplicating the viruses—becoming virus factories—and usually destroying themselves in the process. One idea gaining currency among tumor virologists at the time was that when some viruses infiltrated cells they, in effect, deconstructed themselves. They slipped off their protein coats and then integrated their naked genetic material into the genome of the host cell. They were apparently harmless stowaways; for a long time nothing sinister happened. But then, perhaps when the changed genome was exposed to adverse conditions such as a diminished supply of nutrients or the presence of dangerous chemicals, the cells began replicating wildly. In other words, cancer was the result.

If viruses did alter cells in this way, you might very well find the engine of transformation—their genetic material—lurking in the cancerous cells they created. Zur Hausen told the group that was why his colleague, Heinrich Schulte-Holthausen, had looked for herpes DNA in cervical cancer samples. But tests on almost a hundred cervical cancer biopsies produced only negative outcomes. If these results held up under scrutiny, it meant that women could develop cervical cancer without a previous herpes infection.

Zur Hausen was sure his findings had to be taken seriously. He explained that he had used the same methods to look for Epstein-Barr virus DNA in Burkitt's lymphoma as well as in cancers of the nasopharynx (the uppermost part of the throat). With these techniques, he found cells loaded with complete viral genomes—proof that the methods worked. Zur Hausen had no doubt that an infectious cause for cervical cancer would be found, but he had another candidate in mind. As he began to argue in favor of his alternative, he had the sinking feeling that his remarks might fall flat. Still, he persisted. He had come to Florida with the intention of describing the new direction his research was taking, and he wasn't going to leave without mentioning it. He plowed ahead.

Zur Hausen said that there was a carcinogenic virus which medical researchers had been ignoring. This was the human papillomavirus (HPV). (The word derives from "pap," meaning "nipple," and "oma," meaning "growth." A papilloma is a nipple-like protuberance.) The virus, which attacks the skin as well as mucous membranes, causes warts in many animals. In cows, warts can grow to the size of a human fist and weigh half a pound. Papillomaviruses infected some cottontail rabbits in the American Southwest and produced those unusual hornlike growths on their heads. Warts can turn cancerous in rabbits, cows, and sheep. To be sure, in humans, they are generally benign, a nuisance more than anything else. Medical researchers probably disregarded them for that reason. However, zur Hausen had reports going back a hundred years in which genital warts sometimes became malignant in people. He thought what he had uncovered so far provided a justification for exploring a new tack.

Zur Hausen waited. Surely he would get a hearing, arouse some interest at least. But to his audience, his suggestion was both unexpected and unwelcome. No one had been thinking about the wart virus. The proposal seemed bizarre. The reaction was silence. Profound, stony silence. How could this be? Nothing at all? Zur Hausen looked at the people seated around the room. He knew most of them personally. There was Werner Henle, his former boss, from his fellowship days in Philadelphia. He had spent three and half years working in his lab. They had discussed many scientific questions and even published several research papers together. There was George Klein, a cell biologist from Sweden, who had provided him with biological samples for some of his Epstein-Barr research and who had also collaborated with him on a paper, recently published in *Nature*. Andy Nahmias, a pediatrician from Atlanta and a keen virologist, was a friend. Why weren't they giving his ideas a proper airing, due consideration?[3]

Finally Bernard Roizman got up to respond. He was a forty-three-year-old virologist, born in Romania and educated in the United States. A professor at the University of Chicago, he had been studying herpes for about a decade. The pathogen intrigued him because of its ability to initiate an infection and then remain latent—sometimes for many years.[4] Confident and highly respected, Roizman probably knew more about herpesviruses than anyone else. Roizman told the group that the assays zur Hausen mentioned weren't sensitive enough to pick up a fragment of herpesvirus DNA. He dismissed them as of limited value.[5]

Bernard Roizman went on to report on his own work. He was well poised to take advantage of the groundswell in interest in herpes, and he created a lot of buzz with his investigations, both inside and outside the scientific community. A month before the Key Biscayne meeting, the *New York Times* published a story about him titled "A New Virus Link with Cancer Seen."[6] Zur Hausen had not seen the story, and what Roizman said came as a complete surprise. In his slightly accented English, Roizman addressed the conference. The room was hushed as everyone paid attention. Roizman had important news. He had actually found a fragment of herpes DNA in a cervical cancer specimen. He had detected the fingerprint at the scene of a crime—and said that to his knowledge he was the first person to have done this. It was a remarkable positive result. Zur Hausen could see by the nods and smiles of the people around him that it quickly eclipsed his own negative findings.

Viruses are so small that it wasn't until 1939 that anyone actually saw one with an electron microscope. After that, researchers discovered they came in myriad shapes. Some (like herpesviruses) resembled soccer balls; others looked like filaments, blobs, or bullets. Many had spikes sticking out of them. Scientists could use their distinctive appearance to identify them. However, when viruses hid in the genome of their hosts, they were invisible to an electron microscope. Their camouflage would be complete were it not for the fact that biochemical methods to sequence nucleic acid were being developed. Even if the virus could not be seen, its genetic material could be detected. Still in their infancy in 1972, the methods for doing this were cumbersome, slow, and not perfectly reliable. It was not difficult for the scientists in the room to attribute zur Hausen's results to an imperfect technique—to conclude that Roizman's methodology was better and his data more trustworthy.

Later everyone milled around the coffee urn, often a time when the real communication began. The discussion returned to the subject of Roizman's presentation. Zur Hausen asked Roizman if he expected to find only *fragments* of herpes DNA in cervical biopsies. It was quite possible, the distinguished virologist said. Zur Hausen was skeptical about this, in part, because it meant supposing that the herpesvirus was quite different from other cancer-causing viruses (which left whole genomes in the tumors they created). He didn't express this concern, but did ask Roizman whether he could have a sample from the tumor he had been investigating. That would allow him to test the sensitivity of his methods. (Roizman promised to send him one, but nothing ever arrived in his lab in Erlangen.)

During the break, no one referred to zur Hausen's proposal for a new direction research might take. Suddenly he was an outsider. It was an unusual feeling for the scientist who had moved up remarkably quickly in the ranks of German academia and had published numerous research papers in prestigious journals. He had not anticipated convincing everyone that his approach was the correct one right away. But he did think people who knew him would respect the fact that he did not reach conclusions lightly. He expected them to find his ideas worth considering. When I spoke to zur Hausen about the meeting in Florida, he admitted, "It was a low point. I didn't find any credibility for my suggestions."

Paradigms die hard, as Thomas Kuhn famously observed in *The Structure of Scientific Revolutions*: "Novelty only emerges with difficulty, manifested by resistance, against a background provided by expectation."[7] Scientists do not give up working theories at the first sign of difficulty. Indeed, they may not recognize that first sign *as* a difficulty. When I reached Bernard Roizman by phone at his Chicago office, to ask him how zur Hausen's suggestions about the papillomavirus struck him at the meeting in Florida, I was startled by his response. He said, "Actually my understanding was that his proposal came much later. I cannot pinpoint this. You have to remember the context of the time. There were a large number of proposals about viruses causing cancer. It was just one more virus. When somebody gets up at a meeting and says; 'I believe that virus X causes cancer,' it's not likely to have an impact unless he shows some data. I think his suggestion came later. For some reason, 1978 sticks in my mind."

Intrigued by this divergence from zur Hausen's own perception, I decided to call some of the other participants from the meeting as well. I spoke to Dr. Andre Nahmias in Atlanta, and we had a long phone conversation about many topics, including his passion for prevention of disease. Nahmias told me that he started to research herpes early on in his practice, when he was asked to treat a baby with the condition. He showed that babies could inherit it from their mothers—an unexpected finding at the time. In the sixties and seventies, he suggested that genital herpes could be a cause of cervical cancer. I learned that Nahmias also thought zur Hausen didn't come out publically in favor of HPV until many years after the Florida symposium. "In 1980, I was organizing a big meeting about human herpesviruses in Atlanta. The hypothesis then was herpes and cervical cancer. Many more data were obtained that were suggestive, although causality is very difficult to prove. I invited Harald to come and speak. I think it was his first talk on papilloma in an international meeting. Actually because the fad was strong, he was careful to say, 'Well, it could be the papilloma *and* herpes.'"

Finally, I rang up George Klein in Stockholm. It was late in the evening for him, but we chatted for awhile, mostly about the tenacity of the idea that genital herpes was the cause of cervical cancer—or, as he put it, "the almost desperate effort of the herpes simplex virologists to keep the notion that herpes simplex 2 was the causative agent of cervical carcinoma." He said, "It was a very interesting sociological phenomenon. I have seen it happening in other fields. A very large part of even the good work of herpes simplex virologists was supported by cancer funds. They were trying to defend the herpes simplex etiology. Whether conscious or not, they were clearly defending it, because that is what their support depended on. The moment herpes simplex was not interesting for cancer, the supporting funds from cancer would disappear." And as for HPV? "My memory," he told me, "is that zur Hausen did not come forward at this time for HPV, but came forward very strongly in critically examining the evidence for herpes simplex and tearing it to pieces."

What accounts for this Rashomon effect? (The phenomenon is named after an Akira Kurosawa film in which the characters all have radically different recollections of a dramatic event.) One reason for the differing memories may be that nothing about zur Hausen's suggestion appeared in print right away. As he wrote to me in an email, "Indeed, the publication of the reports in *Cancer Research* took an enormously long period of time. Upon request by the organizers, I separated the articles on all negative findings of herpes simplex viruses, and also on the suspicion that Condylomata Acuminata [genital warts] may play a role in cervical cancer." An article about the negative findings regarding herpes came out in 1974[8] and one about human papillomavirus and cervical cancer in 1976.[9] I also wondered whether Zur Hausen's idea was simply too new. Perhaps it did not really register with his listeners and they promptly forgot it. As Kuhn writes, "Initially, only the anticipated and usual are experienced even under circumstances where anomaly is later observed. Further acquaintance, however, does result in awareness of something wrong or does relate the effect to something that has gone wrong before. That awareness of anomaly opens a period in which conceptual categories are adjusted until the initially anomalous has become the anticipated."[10]

The disappointing reception for zur Hausen's idea did have one good outcome. As he later wrote, "There was less competition for us to worry about; afterwards hardly any researcher dealt with papillomaviruses and cancer."[11] Zur Hausen was confident that he was right, but he knew that proving it would involve a major research effort and new ways of thinking. Unlike some other pathogens, HPV is species-specific. The form which infects humans doesn't affect animals and vice versa. (Influenzas are, for instance, quite different; they cross species barriers. Some flus whose normal hosts are pigs or birds can also infect humans. This is why the H1N1 "swine flu" recently caused such consternation. It is also why flu vaccines can be tested in ferrets or mice.) Zur Hausen had no animals he could use for HPV experiments. And human subjects were out of the question because of the risk of cancer.[12] Adding to the difficulty, papillomaviruses, unlike herpesviruses, could not be cultured in the lab.[13] This made more experiments impossible. The celebrated Prussian physician, Robert Koch, articulated a set of postulates which specified when a microorganism caused a disease. One of the most important of these required isolating a pathogen from a sick animal, growing it in a lab, and then injecting it into a healthy creature. If that animal got sick, the microorganism was to blame. But this research avenue was blocked. Not only did the wart virus pose significant technical difficulties, it also posed theoretical ones. Koch's postulates had served scientists very well, but how was causality to be established when it was impossible to fulfill all of his criteria?

To indict HPV, new tools were needed. Part of the answer lay with the genetic probe that zur Hausen and scientists such as Roizman had just begun to use. A probe for human papillomavirus DNA could be created and then used to tease matching DNA from cervical tissue. But as it turned out, barriers littered even this way forward. Perhaps it was just as well, but zur Hausen did not know that for almost ten years, this technique would fail him. He would not find papillomavirus DNA where he thought it ought to be. Reaching his goal would take extraordinary perseverance.

The conference in Key Biscayne ended on December 10, the day Apollo 17's landing module docked on the moon. As the scientists crossed back over the drawbridge to the Florida mainland, zur Hausen was still certain his ideas had merit. He was determined to proceed. The fact that he was bucking a popular trend did not deter him. He returned to Germany, optimistic about overcoming the hurdles ahead of him. He told me, "I must confess I was really convinced I was on the right track." All he had to do was prove it.

HE COULD ENTERTAIN HIMSELF FOR HOURS IN THE FOREST OR THE MARSH

The day I met Harald zur Hausen, winter was starting in Heidelberg. As I walked from my hotel to the *Deutsches Krebsforschungszentrum* (DKFZ)—the "German Cancer Research Center"—cold sleety rain was falling, and a thick mist hung over the Neckar River, which bisected the town. Professor zur Hausen had been the scientific director of the center for twenty years. He became a professor emeritus in 2003, but still kept an office in the Applied Tumor Virology Building. Just off the lobby, I found a plain white door that had a small sign with his name on it. A printed notice directed visitors to report next door. I knocked on another plain white door, and zur Hausen's secretary, Lisa Braun-Krieling ushered me in. "I'm early," I said apologetically. "That's fine," she said. "He likes that." (Later I discovered that zur Hausen is famous for his insistence on punctuality.)

I passed a desk covered with mountains of thick folders. "His correspondence," Braun-Krieling said with a smile. In the office, large windows overlooked a busy courtyard. The DKFZ is a National Research Center, located on the University of Heidelberg campus, and outside I could see students, many of whom were riding bikes despite the inclement weather, rushing to class. Several large colored photographs of lions, elephants, and other animals occupied one wall of the office. "My wife is from South Africa," zur Hausen told me, gesturing at the pictures, "we try to visit at least once a year. I am an enthusiastic wildlife photographer."

We sat at a small table. I pulled out my tape recorder, and Braun-Krieling brought us coffee. Zur Hausen, who has thick white hair and piercingly blue eyes, was wearing a tweed jacket and a green silk tie. He spoke quickly, eager to impart as much information as he could in the time we had. I was hoping to find out more about how his research had unfolded and also gain some insights into the kind of person he is. What were the early influences on a man who helped to launch a medical revolution? Our conversation was wide-ranging, touching on his family, cancer, viruses, and conviction—his sense that he was getting somewhere, though for many years others could not see it. Zur Hausen was friendly and polite. He has a serious manner, but I discovered that he has a dry sense of humor. He told me that his brothers, with whom I had arranged interviews, had called him up. They were worried about these interviews, he said. He laughed, "They asked me, 'What do we have to say?' I said, 'Anything you like!'"

After an hour and a half, my time was up; zur Hausen had another appointment. A car was waiting. I walked back across the Neckar River to my hotel. Over the next few days, I talked to some of zur Hausen's colleagues in Heidelberg and elsewhere. I travelled south to Munich, east to Jena, to what was formerly East Germany, and west to a couple of small towns in the Ruhr. After ten days I flew home, my mind buzzing with impressions and new ideas.

Harald zur Hausen was the youngest in his family. When he was born in 1936, his sister, Eleonore, was three, his brother, Winfried, was six, and his eldest brother, Manfred, was nine. When I asked zur Hausen what his parents, Eduard and Melanie, were like, he said, "They were very pleasant people from my point of view." Eduard was kindly and generous. He never spoke harshly to his children and also didn't believe in corporal punishment, an unusual point of view at the time.

The zur Hausens lived in the northern Ruhr, a part of Germany in which the family had deep roots. Harald's great grandfather, Theodor, had owned a large estate, zur Hausen's Hof, in Gladbeck. A giant of a man, he stood almost two meters tall and had eighteen children. He was successful enough to be able to rent a castle in which to live—Schloss Wittringen. But his wealth did not survive intact into the next generation, as the inheritance was parceled out eighteen different ways. Harald's grandfather, August, farmed and operated a sawmill in a small place called Resse, not far from Gladbeck.

Harald's father, Eduard, studied agronomy, but the First World War, in which he served as an officer, interrupted his education, and he never returned to it. After the 1918 Armistice, Eduard joined a brigade of German soldiers (known as the Freikorps) who volunteered to fight the Bolsheviks in Latvia. In 1919, while stationed in Riga, Eduard met Melanie. She was the daughter of a factory manager—an accomplished pianist who had studied at the Conservatory in Riga, a great gardener, and a wonderful cook. A month later, the two married, and they soon moved to Germany. They settled for awhile in Bavaria, but eventually made their home back in the Ruhr, in Gelsenkirchen, a town of about 300,000, where Eduard worked with his father in the sawmill business.

Eduard took a keen interest in new scientific and technological developments. For several years in the thirties, his hobby was ballooning. This was when Germany was pioneering lighter-than-air craft, and the airships, the *Graf Zeppelin* and the *Hindenburg*, operated regular transatlantic flights from Germany to North America and Brazil. Eduard got a pilot's license and on Sunday afternoons, when the weather was fine, enjoyed taking friends for balloon rides. He liked watching the toy landscape unfolding below, the tiny houses, the miniature trains, the postage-stamp-sized fields. It was wonderfully quiet, the only sounds the occasional crowing of a cock or barking of a dog. To be sure, he experienced some close calls. Once, a young man who was helping to hold down the balloon while it was being filled with gas didn't let go in time. He was carried aloft and midair had to clamber *up* his rope into the balloon's basket. Another time, Eduard was caught in a thunderstorm. The thunderhead sucked him almost 1,000 feet skyward and then a downdraft plunged him back to the ground. He managed to avoid crashing by throwing all the ballast overboard and came to earth safely, narrowly missing a factory smokestack. This mishap didn't deter him from going ballooning again. The Second World War, however, put a stop to all such pleasures. The European skies would not be quiet again for a long time.

When war broke out in September of 1939, Eduard was called up to enlist—despite the fact that he was fifty and had already served his country once in the First World War. That left Melanie to take care of the four children—her youngest, Harald, only three at the time. Gelsenkirchen was an obvious target for the Allies because of its collieries and oil refinery. The RAF first attacked on the night of May 14, 1940, and throughout the war came back again and again. In 1943, during the Battle of the Ruhr, the air raids were particularly intense as the Allies increased their efforts to undermine Germany's industrial capacity and its ability to wage war. On the night of June 25, 1943, 473 RAF bombers hit Gelsenkirchen and two weeks later, another 418 planes returned.

Harald zur Hausen's brother, Winfried, remembered those days vividly. I visited him at his home in Krefeld, also in the Ruhr. He is a retired landscape architect, the author of ten books about gardening, and a painter. He is a cheerful man with a whimsical outlook, and his house was filled with art, sculptures, masks, paintings, and pottery. Portraits of his family hung on one wall of the living room. Among them were two oil paintings of chimpanzees. When I asked him if those were his, he flashed a mischievous grin. He said, "I thought if we are going to have an *Ahnen* [forefathers'] gallery, they belong; they are the ancestors." Over lunch, in a mixture of German and English, he spoke about the past:

> The nights with the bombs were horrible. Every night we had to take Harald, when he was very young, and my sister, and we had to go into the cellar or to a nearby school where there was a bigger cellar. I took Harald and my mother took my sister. Always bombs and bombs and bombs. We listened to a military radio station. My elder brother was a *Flakhelfer* [an assistant with the anti-aircraft defense].

> They had to go at the age of fifteen. He knew the direction of the airplanes. It was a secret, but he told us. He knew how to do it and he told us what was coming.

Harald began going to primary school in 1942, but within a few months the school closed because of the bombing raids. Schools did not reopen until the war ended. Melanie sent Harald and Eleonore to their Aunt Dora, a teacher who lived on a farm in Coesfeld, near Münster. She thought the children would be safer there, and, also important, that they would be able to go to Dora's school. They did attend, but Harald said they didn't learn much. "Basically we were not very interested in school at this time." Winfried was older, so the *Kinderlandverschickung*, a government evacuation program for children, took him away from the industrial heartland. Along with his schoolmates, he went to Bad Reichenhall, a spa town in Bavaria near the Austrian border.

In 1944, Eduard, who was on the Russian front, suffered a serious heart attack. "That was luck," said Harald zur Hausen. "He was released from the military service completely. It was the same time that the attack on Hitler took place, on the 27th of July, and the Nazi government tried to get rid of the old officers. They didn't trust them." Lieutenant-Colonel Claus von Stauffenberg, a decorated veteran of the Afrika Korps campaign, had attempted to kill Hitler with a briefcase bomb. Members of Hitler's inner circle suspected longtime officers of not supporting Nazi ideals. They expelled hundreds from the army and executed dozens. By this time, Eduard was safely out of the turmoil.

In 1945, as the German Wehrmacht was collapsing in the face of the Allied advance, Eduard grew anxious about the safety of the children. He brought his three youngest to a rural area south of Bremen. Harald was in one village, Winfried and Eleonore in another. Although this part of Germany also suffered from heavy bombardments, the children were not hurt. Meanwhile, Manfred was a prisoner of war, in custody of the Americans. In June, they turned him over to the Russians. While on a forced march through Czechoslovakia, he escaped by slipping away into a grainfield. After walking west for nine nights, he crossed the border into Germany under cover of darkness.

Remarkably, the zur Hausens all survived the war. By the end of 1945, they were back in Gelsenkirchen, where they began putting the war years behind them and picking up the pieces of their lives again.

Their town was a ruined shell. Three-quarters of the buildings were reduced to rubble. The zur Hausen home was also damaged —by a German bomb destined for London that went astray and landed about a hundred meters away. Though the house still stood, the windows were shattered. Looters had stolen many family treasures, including photographs. For the young people, the priority was school—making up for lost time. Harald's aunt ensured that when he enrolled in school, he started in grade 4, despite having missed most of what came before. Harald described himself as an "average" pupil. When he was ten, he entered the local gymnasium (a secondary school for students heading toward an academic stream). "The first year was difficult," he said, "I had so much catching up to do."

Winfried thought that the reputation for being troublemakers that he and his elder brother, Manfred, had acquired didn't help:

> My elder brother had done much nonsense at school and I, too, had struggled with the teachers. I think they didn't understand us; the teachers we had at the time were old—and old-fashioned. When Harald came to the same school, the classroom teacher read his name and burst out, "*Wieviel kommen denn noch von der Sorte?*" [How many more of this type are coming?] Harald didn't know what he meant. He was very perplexed.

Although Harald's teachers allowed him to pass to the next grade at the end of the first year, they had great reservations. "My teachers didn't think I would make it," Harald recalled laughingly.

But Harald *was* learning; his home was in the countryside, on the outskirts of Gelsenkirchen, so the fields and farms nearby were his classroom. He became profoundly curious about the natural world. When he was about eight, he got a notebook, put his name on the cover, and below that wrote "scientist." He used the book to record his observations of birds and animals. Winfried remembered him describing how a cuckoo laid its egg in another bird's nest and, later, how the young cuckoo ejected the other nestlings. "I would have been inclined to interfere," said Winfried, "but Harald just wanted to see what happened."

Harald developed a lifelong friendship with Heinrich Schulte-Holthausen, a boy of the same age who lived on a neighboring farm and shared his passion for birds. Schulte-Holthausen was not only one of

Harald's oldest friends, but he was also one of his earliest scientific collaborators. (He was the one who helped him look at whether herpes simplex type 2 was a possible cause of cervical cancer. Their negative findings on this score opened the door for another hypothesis.) Schulte-Holthausen became a professor in the Institute of Molecular Biology at the University of Essen, where I reached him by phone. He told me that as boys he and Harald roamed freely through the meadows and woods surrounding their homes. They knew where the birds nested and learned their habits. They scoured the countryside for tiny lizards and kept them in a terrarium which his father gave him. "All the other boys in our class, who were living in town, went to sporting events. But for us, it took at least forty-five minutes to get there, and we had no bicycles. We had to go by foot," Schulte-Holthausen said. So instead of playing soccer, they played in the woods. "We were both lucky in a sense because my parents supported me and his parents supported him. It was an environment in which nobody inhibited us, nobody laughed at us." While their parents encouraged them to follow their enthusiasms, they didn't participate or try to direct them. Schulte-Holthausen said, "My father was a farmer; he was not the man to play with us children."

Schulte-Holthausen and zur Hausen were both bookish, although for a period after the war, books were hard to come by. "So I copied a book, by hand, like a medieval monk," Schulte-Holthausen said, chuckling at the memory. For his part, zur Hausen memorized the Latin names of birds. Schulte-Holthausen recalled, "At a very young age, Harald was already an ornithologist. One day he told me, 'I know the Latin name of every European bird.' He said, 'Just ask me.' He was probably eleven or so." I asked Schulte-Holthausen whether zur Hausen was particularly studious, but he said, "Oh no, we were boys like any other boys. I never thought Harald was very different. We played together, we had fun together."

But all the while, zur Hausen was honing his powers of careful observation. When he was about twelve, he wrote a description of how, on a winter's day, a small Siberian hawk attacked a duck, trying to kill it. The attempt was unsuccessful, but zur Hausen thought it was noteworthy, and his short piece about it appeared in a German hunting journal, *Wild und Hund*. It was his first publication. At the same time, zur Hausen began reading about medical researchers. A biography of Robert Koch, the German doctor who found the cause of both anthrax and tuberculosis, deeply impressed him. It wasn't a book, strictly speaking, more of a pamphlet. Still it made such an impact that to this day, zur Hausen remembers the imprint, "Lux-Jugend-Lesebogen." Zur Hausen told me that he was intrigued by Koch's "persistence and the ingenuity with which he developed his techniques." The idea of detecting the cause of a disease appealed to him greatly. He said, "I was fascinated by the discovery of tuberculosis, which was not recognized by many physicians of the time as an infectious disease." In 1882, when Koch announced that he had found what produced this illness, most doctors believed that miasma, bad or noxious air, was responsible, an idea popular since Roman times.

At fourteen, zur Hausen moved with his parents and his sister to Vechta, a small town in the north of Germany; his father had a job in Oldenburg, managing pest control on farms. Zur Hausen's two brothers remained in Gelsenkirchen. Vechta was even more rural than Gelsenkirchen. Deer and foxes as well as a host of small animals lived in a forest nearby, and a great marsh provided habitat for many species of birds. Schulte-Holthausen often visited, and together they explored the countryside looking for birds just as they had in Gelsenkirchen.

Manfred zur Hausen and his wife Doris live in Schermbeck, also in the northern Ruhr. Manfred returned to university, got his PhD in chemistry, and worked for Huels AG as a chemist, eventually becoming the director of production. He retired several years ago. I visited the zur Hausens' comfortable home, and while drinking coffee and sampling Doris's *Weihnachtsgebaeck* (Christmas cookies), we chatted. Manfred described Harald this way:

> He was curious, interested in the world around him. He was mostly in the fields, in the marsh, in the woods. He found squirrels, and raised them. He found snakes. When he took us onto the marsh, and he heard the bird calls, he could tell us their names. He wanted to know everything—the fundamentals. He wanted to observe everything, also the flora. He was an exceptional nature lover. He could entertain himself for hours in the forest or the marsh.

Once Harald found a dead fox, decapitated it, and asked his mother to boil the head so that he could have the skull, teeth and all. He liked to keep it on his desk. When he found a dead mole, he painstakingly dissected the small creature, documenting everything he found. He also taught himself a lot about mushrooms. Like his later endeavors, this involved experiments that did not always work out. Winfried recalled, "He studied mushrooms and he brought them home and we cooked them and ate them. Once he got a toadstool, but it looked like a *Steinpilz*, a good mushroom. My mother cooked it and the water became bluish. We tried to eat it but it was impossible; it was not edible."

Harald's mother was extraordinarily sympathetic to his curiosity, perhaps because she, too, was intrigued by many aspects of the world around her. Said Winfried, "My mother was very interested in medicine. We didn't go to doctors often; she was able to take care of us. We had a wonderful garden, with all the tulips and all the flowers. She liked to try out new plants, not the usual plants. She was an *Alleskenner* [a polymath]."

At the gymnasium in Vechta, Harald started to earn excellent grades. He read widely in a number of scientific fields, but especially medicine. He was also forming a distaste for orthodoxy, for dogma that was maintained in the absence of evidence. He became increasingly skeptical about religion and told his religion teacher so. He had no hesitation about confronting an authority or going against a received opinion:

> I began gradually to become a disbeliever. I was particularly annoyed about some of the statements which he [the teacher] made frequently. He would tell us, "You just have to believe. Even if you can't explain it, it's just a question of belief." I hated these types of statements. The teacher suffered very much during this period of time, because there was one other pupil in my class and the two of us brought him into painful situations, always asking him why and so on. In the end, he was helpless and just said, "You have to believe."

Zur Hausen described himself as a "confessing nonbeliever." While still the scientific director of the DKFZ, he wrote a book called *Genome und Glaube: der Unsichbare Käfig* (Genomics and Belief: The Invisible Cage). It was about the intersection of our understanding of genetics and religion.[14] It was published in 2003, but zur Hausen thought the topic was so important that he recently began working on a revised edition.

> I wanted to point out some of the difficulties that exist between belief, particularly Christian belief because I am more familiar with

> that one, less so with other religions, and the advances of science. As the history of people like Giodarno Bruno and Galileo shows, this type of conflict has existed for a long period of time. My final conclusion was basically that we should not have an absolutely fixed opinion about things. I called it "dynamic rationalism." We should be anti-dogmatic, really. That was my main message.

In the final years of school, as Harald was learning more about science, it became crystal clear what he wanted to do. He never had any doubts. When he was sixteen, he announced his intentions to his brother, Manfred, who was visiting Vechta with Doris, then his girlfriend. Harald said, "I'm going to study medicine and become a researcher. Then I will get the Nobel Prize and invite you all to Stockholm." Manfred commemorated the event with a photograph of Harald and Doris, his arms over her shoulders. He sent his picture, on which he wrote, "The Future Nobel Prize Winner," to Winfried.

It would take another fifty-six years for Harald's prediction to come true. And then indeed, he would win the Nobel Prize and invite his family to the festivities in Sweden. Doris told me, "When he invited us, we said, 'We'd like to come, we're happy to come.' And we reminded him that he had thought about it, years ago."

A POSSIBLE RELATIONSHIP BETWEEN PAPILLOMAVIRUSES AND CANCER

Harald zur Hausen frowned as he sipped his coffee. "It was horrible," he said, remembering the double major he chose when he enrolled at the University of Bonn in 1955—biology and medicine. Biology turned out to be a disastrous choice for him. "You had to draw the mandibles of insects, which really didn't bring you any further ahead. Molecular biology was not being taught. I gave it up after seven semesters and then I studied only medicine."

When I asked zur Hausen how he came to his core idea—that viruses might play a role in human cancer—he said, "It was during my time as a student, because I learned about bacteriophages." Often called "phages" for short, they are viruses that can infect and destroy bacteria. Later when I read about them, I learned that these small entities were remarkably instructive. Solving the mysteries of their behavior has revealed many important biological processes. Their story began in Agra, India, in the late nineteenth century with an Englishman, Ernest Hanbury Hankin. He was working as a government bacteriologist at a time when most European authorities thought that the Ganges spread disease, particularly cholera. Ancient Hindu tradition held the contrary—that the Ganges was sacred and had healing powers. Hankin showed that these ideas were not mere folklore; they had a scientifically demonstrable basis. In fact, the Ganges did not spread cholera; it was remarkably free of microbes. Something in the sacred water was killing them. The Pasteur Institute in Paris published Hankin's findings, but he did not study the phenomenon any further.[15] He was interested in many subjects—among other things he published a pioneering work on the flight patterns of pterodactyls and an article about the geometric patterns in Islamic art.

The story of bacteriophages continued in 1915, when Frederick Twort, another British scientist, found small agents that destroyed bacteria.[16] Two years later, a French Canadian bacteriologist, Felix d'Hérelle, made the same discovery. Twort wasn't certain what he had come across, but d'Hérelle appreciated it right away. He was a self-taught scientist, a colorful adventurer who travelled all over the world. For a time, he was a professor at Yale, and then Joseph Stalin invited him to work at Tblisi Institute in Georgia. (He had to flee for his life when a friend of his fell in love with the mistress of Lavrenty Beria, the head of the secret police.[17]) D'Hérelle confidently asserted that he had found "an invisible microbe that is antagonistic to the dysentery bacillus."[18] He coined the name of the pathogen from the word "bacteria" and a Greek word, *phagein*, meaning "to eat."[19] Bacteriophages are the most widely distributed biological entity on earth; millions of them populate every grain of dirt and droplet of seawater. In appearance, they resemble lunar landing modules, with spiky tails that help them penetrate the outer membranes of bacteria. They possess many genes found nowhere else.

The tale unfolded further in 1921 when Jules Bordet and Mihai Ciucu at the Pasteur Institute in Brussels made a surprising observation: bacteria sometimes seemed to spontaneously generate bacteriophages. But how and why did they do this? Did bacteria contain within themselves the seeds of their own destruction? The puzzle took many years to solve. Bordet grasped the essence of the solution early on, when he wrote, "The faculty to produce bacteriophages is inscribed in the heredity of the bacterium."[20]

More of the account came out after World War II, as a result of Andre Lwoff's experiments. He was a French Jew of Russian extraction who joined the resistance and hid American pilots in his apartment after they had been shot down in Nazi territory. Following the war, Lwoff received the Resistance Medal and was made a commander of the Legion of Honor for his bravery. His study of bacteriophages earned him another major award—the Nobel. Lwoff knew that phages infecting a bacterium usually multiply rapidly and quickly destroy it in the process. But they can also act insidiously and slowly, and in a series of carefully designed experiments he explained how this happened. By growing individual bacteria and then letting them divide, he demonstrated that after infection, they can multiply for successive generations without showing any apparent problems or producing any phages. However, when a triggering event occurs, such as exposure to UV radiation, viruses spill out of the host bacterium. A latent form of the bacteriophage, which Lwoff called a "prophage," becomes integrated in the genome of a host cell and replicates along with the bacteria.[21] Phages showed how a virus could hide out among a host cell's genes, where it acted like a ticking time bomb—something that fascinated zur Hausen.

In the 1920s and 1930s, researchers studied bacteriophages extensively. Lacking other antibiotics, scientists thought these tiny antimicrobial entities might be useful therapeutic agents. Zur Hausen, however, was intrigued with the way they hijacked the reproductive machinery of the bacteria they infected. If phages could infiltrate the genome of their hosts, maybe other viruses that attacked humans could do the same. "I thought this might be an answer to human cancers," zur Hausen told me. "I was deeply and profoundly interested in the question of whether cancer had anything to do with viral infections. I wondered whether it might be due to the cells' uptake of novel genetic materials from those agents and their persistence in the cells."

Zur Hausen has a well-deserved reputation for persistence and focus. However, his start in medicine was not exactly straight arrow, and several years would elapse before he could work on the questions that intrigued him so much. In 1957 he left the University of Bonn for the Bernhard Nocht Institute for Maritime and Tropical Diseases at the University of Hamburg—Germany's most important research center for the subject. "I was interested in tropical medicine because I was interested in infections," zur Hausen said. But he ran into problems when it came to a topic for his medical thesis, a graduation requirement. In those days, in Germany, the supervising professor set the subject for this exercise. Zur Hausen recounted, "I went to the director of the tropical institute. Could he propose a theme? He said, 'I have this nice colleague who certainly has a very good thing for you.' Then I went to the colleague and told him I wanted to do my medical thesis. He was immediately enthusiastic and said he had something that would be perfect. It was an absolutely stupid project. I saw that there would be no interesting outcome." The thesis would take years and would involve counting amoebic cysts in the stools of monkeys. (Amoebas are parasites that cause a type of dysentery.) Though zur Hausen liked living in Hamburg, a lively city with many cultural activities, he decided to drop the topic and go to the University of Düsseldorf, which also offered courses in tropical medicine.

Zur Hausen remembered, "There was a professor there who had previously worked for the Bayer Company. During his time as director of the lab for parasitology, it developed Atabrine and Resochin, two famous anti-malaria drugs. What I didn't know is that he had told his other colleagues that he had worked long enough and it was now time to become a professor. I went and asked him for a thesis. I got another stupid proposal. I thought to myself, 'I cannot give it up a second time. Now I have to go through with it.'" The topic seemed eccentric, to say the least. He was to study the antiseptic properties of floor waxes—their effect on certain types of bacteria, particularly after UV irradiation. "In the end it was not totally uninteresting. Some data came out," zur Hausen said, and then he smiled. "While I was here in Heidelberg, a student from Düsseldorf arrived to do some research. She told me that at the university, they were digging into the archives and found my thesis. She said, 'We found out that you were working with floor waxes.' I said, 'Yes, I am indeed, *Ein Bona Wax Doktor* [Bona Wax—a popular German brand of floor polish].' She said, 'I will not tell anyone.' I said, 'You can tell everyone!' I found it quite nice that she wanted to be so secretive."

Zur Hausen had been dreaming about becoming a researcher since he was a teenager. After two years of clinical practice, he qualified as a medical doctor in 1962. He secured a position as a research fellow in the Institute of Hygiene and Microbiology at the University of Düsseldorf. At that time, Harald zur Hausen also met a pretty young woman, Elke, who was training to be a medical technician. They married, and a son, Jan Dirk, was born in 1965.

But zur Hausen was not content. Despite his high hopes, the institute turned out to be a disappointment; its atmosphere was stultifying. The organization did routine biodiagnostics and offered little guidance for a young and inexperienced scientist. "When I started to work, I had a number of crazy ideas about what one could theoretically do. I could do what I wanted; they didn't care." Whenever zur Hausen went to the director, Walter Kikuth, and tried to propose something to him, "he would say, in a broad Baltic accent, 'Well, it sounds very good. Why don't you try it?' It was hopeless." As a medical student, zur Hausen had suffered from the wrong supervision, but he was beginning to see that no direction was a problem too.

Zur Hausen was also becoming increasingly aware of a significant gap in his knowledge of molecular biology, then emerging as an important discipline. Just over a decade before, on February 28, 1953, a thirty-six-year-old graduate student, Francis Crick, walked into The Eagle, a Cambridge pub, to celebrate. He and his collaborator, twenty-five-year-old James Watson, a postdoctoral fellow, had unraveled the structure of DNA. Crick told his astonished colleagues, "We have discovered the secret of life!" In April, the two published a paper in *Nature* describing what they had learned. They suggested that DNA looked like a twisted ladder or double helix. The sides of the ladder were made up of alternating sugar and phosphate molecules. Each of the rungs contained two nitrogen bases, either adenine and thymine or cytosine and guanine—A, T, C, and G, for short. "The Molecular Structure of Nucleic Acids" was just nine hundred words long, but it fundamentally changed biology.[22]

It was now possible for scientists to read the book of life, but it was still not easy. The biochemical methods needed to reveal the genetic inheritance of any given organism were just starting to be invented. The Institute of Hygiene and Microbiology at the University of Düsseldorf was in a backwater, far from this development. Zur Hausen felt certain that to make any progress exploring the association between cancer and viruses, new molecular techniques were essential. Staying at the institute would probably mean giving up his goal of finding a viral cause of cancer. "By 1965," he said, "I was desperately looking for another place to go." Salvation came in the form of a letter in a wastepaper basket. An inquiry arrived for Walter Kikuth from the United States asking whether any German Fellow would be available for a research position in Philadelphia. "He asked his colleagues whether anyone was interested," zur Hausen said. "No one was, so the letter ended up in a wastepaper basket. However, he mentioned it to me. I pulled it out of the trash and wrote back."

Soon Werner Henle responded to zur Hausen. He was the director of the Virus Diagnostic Laboratory of the Children's Hospital of Philadelphia. Werner's grandfather, Jakob Henle, was a famous anatomist. He was also Jewish, which is why Werner fled Germany in 1936, shortly after qualifying as a doctor at the University of Heidelberg. A year later, Gertrude Szpingier, also a medical graduate, left Germany to join Werner. They were married the day after her arrival in the United States, and from then on, this powerhouse couple worked closely together and made many major contributions to virology.

Werner Henle told zur Hausen that he and Gertrude planned to visit Heidelberg and suggested a meeting. In June 1965, the three scientists sat down for lunch in the old, elegant Europa Hotel. Gertrude was bursting with the news that Anthony Epstein had recently discovered a new virus. The revelation was so fresh that the microbe didn't even have a name and zur Hausen had never heard of it. The discovery was especially exciting because Epstein had found it in a human tumor. Of course, this wasn't enough to prove that it had caused the cancer, but Gertrude Henle maintained that for those scientists who were interested in establishing that such a connection existed, this new pathogen was the hottest trail to follow.

The Henles began studying the new virus when Epstein wanted another lab to confirm his results. He asked a couple of English virologists if they would like to help, but they weren't interested in what Epstein described as "our unorthodox findings."[23] That's when he turned to the Henles, who were much farther away, but whose scientific reputation was stellar. They jumped at the chance to take on some research which they clearly saw as leading edge. Gertrude Henle told zur Hausen that if he joined them in Philadelphia, he would be working with the new pathogen. (By 1968, it had become known as the Epstein-Barr virus.) Though zur Hausen had some regrets about uprooting his young family and leaving his friends and colleagues in Germany, the lure was great. Suddenly, he would be at the forefront of tumor virology. It was like going from a job on the assembly line to working at NASA.

At the end of 1965, the zur Hausens moved to Philadelphia and took a small apartment on Drexel Hill. At first, zur Hausen was dismayed by the lab, located in an inconvenient building in a run-down section of Philadelphia. In the beginning, he also struggled with English, but was soon swept up in the scientific ferment of the place. In just a few years, the Henles discovered many important facts about the Epstein-Barr virus. They showed that it could "immortalize" white bloods cells—that is, cause them to grow and divide indefinitely. Biologists call cells "immortal" if, provided with nutrients and otherwise normal growing conditions, they never die.

The Henles also found that the virus was very common, even outside of Africa. Since Burkitt's lymphoma, with which it was associated in Africa, was rare elsewhere, it was clear other factors must be involved in causing that malignancy. Perhaps most importantly, together with a young German physician, Volker Diehl, who joined their lab shortly after zur Hausen did, the Henles showed that Epstein-Barr virus did cause an infectious illness common in the developed world—mononucleosis.

Zur Hausen relished his discussions with Werner Henle and the opportunity they gave him to engage in a lively give-and-take. He was often amazed at how much time Henle allowed for this, something which he had never experienced at the institute in Düsseldorf. The debate was real; the two men did not always agree. One point on which their scientific intuitions diverged was how the Epstein-Barr virus might cause cancer.

Henle had a strong conviction that the pathogen remained as an intact virus in the cells, causing a persistent infection which eventually led to cancer. This ran squarely against zur Hausen's hunch that it acted like a phage, insinuating its genetic material in the genome of the host cells. Once having done that, its disguise was perfect. It could lurk there for months, even years. It could not be detected by an electron microscope. Eventually, though, the genetic alterations caused the host cells to reproduce in an uncontrolled manner. "Show me," said Henle.[24]

For zur Hausen to prove that he was right, he had to show that even lymphoma cells which contained no visible Epstein-Barr viruses nonetheless contained their DNA. He knew there were techniques for doing this and thought that with the help of the equipment and experts at the Wistar Institute in Philadelphia, he could learn them. Henle generously agreed to let him contact the institute and do some research there. Founded in 1892, it was the first independent biomedical research facility in the United States and by the 1960s was a leader in the development of vaccines and the understanding of cancer. At the institute, zur Hausen met Frantisek Sokol, a wartime refugee from Czechoslovakia. "That was a beautiful relationship we had," zur Hausen said, smiling. "He was an excellent biochemist, very critical. For me he was *the* teacher in molecular biology methodology. He loved to teach me the techniques." From Sokol, he learned how to make a genetic probe, which turned out to be vital for his later discoveries.

A fundamental property of DNA is that it can replicate. When cells divide, new cells need to contain the same genetic information as the old ones. The double helix, the twisted ladder, unwinds; the rungs split, and the single strands are a template for building two new DNA molecules, identical to the original. As Watson and Crick observed, the chemicals which form the rungs always take the same partners. Since A is always paired with T and C with G, the two sides of the ladder are complementary. Scientists can exploit this understanding to see whether a tissue sample contains the DNA of a known virus. First, they isolate the DNA of the virus they have identified. By adding heat and certain chemicals to it, they can split the double strands into single-stranded sequences or probes. To find out if a probe matches a string in a target tissue, researchers extract DNA from the target, unzip it—so that it too is single-stranded—and expose it to the probe. Since complementary segments are attracted to one another, the probe works like bait. If the probe's complement is present, the two will join up. By attaching a radioactive tag to the probe, researchers are able to detect whether a union (often called hybridization) takes place. If it does, the mating leaves a telltale dark spot on a piece of photographic film.

Working with Sokol, zur Hausen became thoroughly familiar with the technique. Could he now find Epstein-Barr virus DNA sequestered in the genome of Burkitt's lymphoma cells? When zur Hausen discussed the question with Sokol, the biochemist pointed out that Burkitt's lymphoma cells contained only a very small number of Epstein-Barr viruses. Because of this, Sokol didn't think hybridization would work. The difficulty was practical, not theoretical, but sometimes the practical looms large in science. Zur Hausen tucked the problem away; he didn't give up, but planned to return to it.

In the meantime, another idea came to him, almost by accident. One day, when zur Hausen was waiting in Henle's office to speak with him, he picked up a copy of the *Bacteriological Review* to pass the time. Browsing through the pages, he was suddenly struck by one article—a review of research about papillomaviruses, known to cause warts in animals and people. He had long thought that the search for carcinogenic pathogens should include papillomaviruses. But little attention was paid to these pathogens, perhaps because they were so familiar, and more of a nuisance than a serious health problem. However, the article indicated that genital warts sometimes turned malignant. Zur Hausen asked Henle if he might borrow the journal; he read and reread the piece. Were the warts linked to cervical cancer?

Zur Hausen did not instantly decide to take up the search for an answer. "People often ask me," he said, 'What was the moment when you had the brilliant idea?' It never happened. It was really a product of careful consideration." Zur Hausen mulled over what he had read and talked about its implications with his friends. Heinrich Schulte-Holthausen, zur Hausen's boyhood companion, remembered those early conversations. While zur Hausen was in Philadelphia, Schulte-Holthausen was studying at Duke University in Durham, North Carolina.

> We met sometimes and then, of course, we spoke about science. He was working on adenoviruses. I was working on the development of cartilage in young chickens. I can remember that he was already talking about a possible relationship between papillomaviruses and cancer. I came very late to tumor virology, but for me the relationship was always self-evident. I never had any doubt. This relationship had already been shown in animal systems. Much was known about the mechanisms.

While zur Hausen was thinking about papillomaviruses and cancer, he was also settling in to life in the United States. In 1967, zur Hausen's second son, Axel, was born. A year later, Henle helped zur Hausen to get a position as assistant professor at the University of Pennsylvania.

Then, unexpectedly, another opportunity presented itself. Eberhard Wecker, who was head of the newly established Virology Institute at the University of Würzburg in northern Bavaria, offered zur Hausen the chance to lead a research group at the institute. He would be able to develop his own program and pick his own colleagues. It didn't take zur Hausen long to decide. He was going back to Germany.

When he said good-bye to Frantisek Sokol, his mentor at the Wistar Institute, he told him that he planned to look for Epstein-Barr DNA in Burkitt's lymphoma cells. Zur Hausen recalled, "He laughed. 'Well, good luck,' he said. He didn't think it was possible."

On a cool blustery day in March 1969, zur Hausen set sail from New York. He had two young sons now, an apartment's worth of furniture purchased in America, and two new hypotheses to test. It was cold when he docked in Bremerhaven, but his boss, Eberhard Wecker, was there to meet him and received him warmly.

GRINDING UP WARTS

One of the first things zur Hausen did when he arrived in Würzburg was hire Heinrich Schulte-Holthausen as his assistant. He'd known Schulte-Holthausen, he told me, "from baby days. We were neighbors and remained close friends." Zur Hausen's boss, Wecker, questioned his choice since Schulte-Holthausen was a chemist, not a virologist. But Zur Hausen assured him he was absolutely the right person for the job.

Though zur Hausen was keen to start studying human papillomaviruses, Schulte-Holthausen was daunted by the prospect. He accepted the thesis that viruses could cause cancer, but he had a concern about the human papillomavirus in particular. Not much was known about it, and there was no way of culturing and growing the pathogen in the lab. Zur Hausen agreed to hold off for the moment. Indeed, there were some other important and interesting questions to investigate.

There was, for example, that unfinished business about Burkitt's lymphoma and Epstein-Barr virus. How did those pathogens cause lymphomas when so few could be seen in the tumors? One possible explanation was that while some cells became cancerous directly when the microbes infected them, others became malignant *indirectly* when pathogens colonized their neighbors. This didn't strike zur Hausen as plausible at all, however. He still thought his original idea was correct—that some of the viruses deposited their DNA in the cellular genome, thereby disrupting its reproductive machinery and turning the cells cancerous. This meant that even those cells in which no viruses could be *seen* were affected by the viral DNA. But could he prove this? Could he find that DNA hidden in the lymphomas?

This was no easy task. Viruses had spent hundreds of thousands of years evolving stratagems to evade the surveillance of the immune system. They were masters of deception. How could zur Hausen ferret them out? First he needed to make a probe for the Epstein-Barr virus. It was not possible to culture the virus in the lab, but zur Hausen devised a clever way around that obstacle. He cultured the *cancer* cells in which a few visible viruses could be found. That gave him a supply of viruses from which he could make a radioactive probe. Then he turned to cancer biopsies in which *no* viruses could be seen. Working together, he and Schulte-Holthausen extracted DNA from these biopsies. They reasoned that if the DNA contained viral as well as cellular material, the two could be separated. Viral DNA is denser than cellular DNA, so it can be detached with a centrifuge, a piece of equipment that separates substances of differing densities by spinning them. Once they had separated the DNA into two components, they introduced the probe to the denser material. By exposing it to something in which the viral DNA was concentrated, they increased the odds of success. The experiment worked like a charm. The probe found its match. The results, which established that Burkitt's lymphoma cells in which no Epstein-Barr viruses were visible could nevertheless contain its DNA, were published in the journal *Nature*.[25] Zur Hausen's hunch that viruses' ability to infiltrate our cellular genome might help to explain the riddle of cancer was beginning to pay off.

Zur Hausen stayed in Würzburg for three years. When another virology institute opened at the University of Erlangen-Nürnberg in southern Bavaria, he was invited to become its chairman. The chance to develop and build an entire organization according to his own lights was a big draw. Zur Hausen was determined that with the move, he would now turn his attention to the human papillomavirus. In the beginning, he said, "I was myself grinding up the warts and purifying the virus." Early on, he realized that the radioactive probes he made from foot warts were not reacting with other skin warts, genital warts, or cervical cancers. Some researchers might have concluded from this that the enterprise was doomed—that foot warts were in no way related to cervical tumors. But zur Hausen interpreted the data differently. He thought it likely that he was dealing with pathogens that were part of the same family, yet genetically distinct. He knew the next step was to characterize these different microbes and their properties. And then he had a fortuitous encounter with a young student, Lutz Gissman, who was working on his diploma—the equivalent of a master's degree in the Anglo-American University tradition.

When I met Gissman in his office, a utilitarian room with white cement walls, he was a professor and the head of the Genome Modifications and Carcinogenesis division in the DKFZ in Heidelberg. He was a wiry man with closely cropped hair and an intense manner. I'd read a little about him before coming and formed the impression of someone who was a technical wizard—a person who was able to conjure usable data from minute quantities of viruses. He told me that he had grown up in Bavaria close to the Austrian border and had gone to a high school that specialized in the humanities. I was surprised to learn that his first intellectual interest was not science, but the Classics—Latin and Greek. He said, "I read a lot. I was interested in philosophy. That was from my language background. I was also very interested in acting." And then he laughed and recalled, "But I must say, fortunately this didn't work out." In his last year of school, Gissman became intrigued by microbiology and decided he would study it in university, while keeping languages "as a hobby." He was at the University of Erlangen when one of his professors told him about a medical researcher called Harald zur Hausen who was going to join the faculty. Zur Hausen was already starting to make a name for himself for his careful and insightful studies of carcinogenic viruses. Gissman immediately thought this was the man with whom he wanted to study. He buttonholed zur Hausen in a hallway soon after he arrived and asked him whether he could do his PhD with him. "He said, 'Yes,' It was a very quick decision," Gissman recalled. "He thinks matters through very thoroughly, but he can also be very spontaneous."

It took awhile for Gissman to finish his diploma, so it wasn't until 1974 that his work with zur Hausen began in earnest. Once it started, he visited a local dermatologist every Friday to collect warts that the physician had removed from his patients' hands and feet. Gissman put them in a thermos bottle filled with liquid nitrogen and raced back to the lab to analyze them. After pulverizing more than three hundred warts, Gissman confirmed that the human papillomaviruses found on the hands and feet were different from those on the genitals. And in fact, by 1976, he and zur Hausen had identified at least four different kinds. The wart family was growing.

Zur Hausen knew that in Germany, it would be difficult to get a good supply of cervical cancer biopsies. For the most part, as in other developed countries, cervical cancer was detected in its early stages in Germany. The tumors were small. Enough tissue was collected for the purposes of diagnosis, but that was all. There wasn't much available for research. But zur Hausen knew that in Africa, the situation was quite different. Cervical cancer was usually detected when the tumor was large. Moreover, genital warts were common as well. He wondered whether a trip to Africa might be a good idea. He talked to Volker Diehl, his colleague from Philadelphia days who had travelled to Kenya in 1968 to gather samples of Burkitt's lymphoma. Diehl was so enthusiastic about zur Hausen's idea, he proposed going with him to get the samples he needed. Supported by a research grant, the two travelled through Kenya and South Africa for three months in the summer of 1976, gathering biopsies as they went. In South Africa, zur Hausen also met a young scientist, Ethel-Michele de Villiers, and toured virology institutes in Pretoria and Johannesburg with her. Later she would join zur Hausen's research group in Germany and, still later, after the breakup of his marriage, would become his second wife.

In early October of 1976, zur Hausen presented his ideas about papillomaviruses and cervical cancer at a meeting of tumor virologists in the Swiss alpine village of Grindelwald. Four years had passed since he had introduced these thoughts to his colleagues in Key Biscayne, Florida. They were still received with skepticism. A Dutch virologist, Peter Bentvelzen, approached him, saying, "What kind of virologist are you? You seem to represent the new branch of speculative virology."[26]

IS THERE SOMETHING NEW?

Despite the difficulties zur Hausen had in changing scientific opinion, his talent for administration was highly regarded. Unexpectedly, the

Institute of Hygiene at the University of Freiburg, at the southwestern tip of Germany, offered him the position of chairman. It was an old organization with a distinguished reputation and it had established relationships with many clinicians. Zur Hausen had a feeling this would be a good place for his research and so in 1977, he moved again. And indeed, here it was, in the lovely old town in the heart of the Black Forest, that his major breakthrough came. Most of the researchers who had been working with zur Hausen in Erlangen followed him and carried on as before. In Freiburg, Lutz Gissman started to investigate genital warts, but soon ran into a problem. He explained, "The amount of virus particles was ten- to one hundred-fold less than in skin warts. I was never able to purify virus from genital warts directly and then extract the DNA from that. We had to use a trick." The trick was first to extract all the DNA, cellular and viral, from the biopsy and then use a centrifuge to separate the denser viral DNA from the lighter cellular one.

In 1981, Ethel-Michele de Villiers arrived in Freiburg as a postdoc. She and Gissman began studying the viral DNA Gissman had obtained from the genital warts. When they cloned and investigated it, they realized it was yet another type, soon called HPV 6. Gissman had high hopes that finally they had found a virus which was also responsible for cervical cancer. Unfortunately, this was not the case. The HPV 6 probe did not match anything in cervical cancer tumors. Later Gissman wrote, "We just had to be patient and investigate more tumors. The thought that Harald zur Hausen's theory could be false never occurred to me."[27]

The way forward involved something Peter Howley discovered. He was then a pathologist at the National Institutes of Health in the US and now is the chairman of the Department of Pathology at Harvard Medical School. He learned how to make genetic probes adhere to sequences that were just partial matches—related but not identical. This seemingly simple innovation turned out to be an extremely useful addition to the biochemist's tool kit. It was all a matter of adjusting the conditions under which a probe was introduced to a target. Howley discovered that probes would join or hybridize with genetic sequences that were similar but not exactly identical if he lowered the temperature and reduced the concentration of the chemicals used in the reaction. Doing this was called creating conditions of low or non-stringency. Raising the temperature and increasing the concentration of the chemical additives made it more likely that the probes would find exact matches. This was called a condition of stringency. The technique was a bit fiddly. "This was an art, in a sense," Gissman explained. "You can imagine the difficulty. You have to adjust the conditions in such a way that similar molecules are picked up, but they [the conditions] are still stringent enough so that you don't have hybridization with everything." With experience, Gissman learned how to hit the Goldilocks zone—get the temperature and chemicals just right for the results he wanted. As you will see, Gissman needed this kind of flexibility for his molecular fishing expeditions.

Another helpful development resulted from what may have seemed like a detour—the investigation of a rare tumor which affected the airway of some children. Associated with papillomaviruses, the tumor was usually not malignant, but it was nevertheless potentially fatal since it could obstruct breathing. Because it resembled a genital wart, zur Hausen thought it would be interesting to test it with an HPV 6 probe. When Gissman did that, under conditions of low stringency, he reeled in the DNA of yet another human papillomavirus—later called HPV 11.

Zur Hausen then decided to ask Matthias Dürst, a PhD student of his, to clone this new viral sequence and see whether *it* might be present in cervical cancers as well as in these airway tumors. Dürst, a Swiss microbiologist, had arrived in Freiburg in October of 1981. Quite quickly, Dürst impressed zur Hausen as being a level-headed and skillful investigator.[28] He had no hesitation about handing over a crucial phase of the investigation to him even though he was relatively new at this type of research. I learned more about Dürst's role when I went to Jena, an old university town in eastern Germany. He was a professor in the Gynecological Department of the Friedrich Schiller University, one of the ten oldest universities in the country.

My arrival in Jena involved a minor adventure. When the train pulled into the station, I attempted to follow the instructions on the door about exiting. I put my hand on a symbol of a palm and waited for the door to open. It didn't. As the train rolled out of the station through the darkness, I figured out what I had done wrong. I had touched the symbol with my gloved hand, when I should have used bare fingers. Fortunately, at the next stop, Naumberg, I was able to get out. It was snowing heavily by then, and there were no taxis in sight. However, I spotted a teen-age girl, talking on a cell phone. When she hung up, I explained what had happened to me and asked her if she would call a cab. "*Kein Problem* [No problem]," she said. Forty Euros later, I was back in Jena, in front of the hotel where I had a reservation. Later reflecting about this, I thought about how sometimes small differences can make *all* the difference. It was certainly true of papilloma research.

Matthias Dürst is a tall, friendly man who speaks flawless English. While I sipped an excellent cup of coffee in his office, he told me that he had lived and studied in England from the time he was thirteen. He said, "I wasn't particularly scientifically oriented, but I was inquisitive." He liked to take things apart, to see how they worked: "My idea was that if something was broken, you could repair it by intuition—a child's attitude, of course." Dürst graduated with a master's in microbiology from the University of Reading and after working in vaccine research for a few years in Switzerland, he decided to go on to a PhD. A colleague, who had studied with zur Hausen, offered to write him a reference letter, so that was how he ended up in Freiburg.

Dürst had been with zur Hausen for less than a year when he set him to work with HPV—under Gissman's watchful eye. The first exciting moment came on a drizzly, dank Friday—November 12, 1982. This was when Dürst discovered that the probe for HPV 11 was related to several sequences in one cervical cancer tumor. The next, even more exciting discovery took place six days later, on November 18, another drizzly day in the Black Forest. Dürst could show that one of the sequences related to HPV 11 bonded with strands from several other known human papillomaviruses under conditions of *low* stringency. But the sequence did not bond with any known HPV types under *stringent* conditions. It was not identical to any of them. The virus was a member of the HPV family, but was new. Furthermore, when Dürst searched for this last fragment in eighteen additional cervical cancer biopsies taken from German patients, he detected a match in eleven (about 60 percent) of them. He immediately told Gissman, and the two men rushed over to see zur Hausen in his office. Their discovery was so fresh that the radiographic film was still dripping with developing fluid when they knocked on his door. Despite his many administrative duties, zur Hausen always had time for his researchers and listened to what they had to say right away. After a few minutes, when he had digested the news, Dürst recalled, "He said, 'This is what we have been looking for.' He went to his cabinet and got a bottle of cognac. This was unusual during the day, at least in Germany. Obviously for him, this was very interesting. He wanted to spontaneously toast the exciting result. For me, I was not so much involved in this history of the whole thing, so I did not take in its implication completely. I was not aware that he had a postulate that was not appreciated by other colleagues—that he was swimming against the stream, so to speak."

Later zur Hausen wrote, "For the rest of the day, it was difficult for me to think about anything else, other than our results, and that night I could hardly sleep."[29] After ten years of searching, zur Hausen had finally found the DNA from a human papillomavirus in a cervical cancer. This did not by itself show that the virus caused the cancer. However, Dürst also discovered that the isolate, soon known as HPV 16, was absent from most benign papillomas. That meant the virus's association with malignancy was not likely a matter of chance.

The next step was to announce the results. "The paper was written very quickly, in a couple of days," said Dürst. "There was real pressure to get it out because others were on it as well. Gerard Orth's laboratory in France was near to cloning this isolate, and some laboratories in the United States were close as well. The paper was published in record time in the *Proceedings for the National Academy of Science*.[30]

This was the major breakthrough, but there was more work to be done. Though Dürst had found HPV 16 in 60 percent of German cervical cancer biopsies, in biopsies from Kenya and Brazil, the pathogen appeared in fewer samples—about 35 percent. Obviously, geography played a role in the incidence of HPV 16 infections—something that needed to be further described and documented. Because HPV 16 did not occur in all cervical cancers, this indicated other varieties had to be sought out and characterized. Zur Hausen asked Michael Boshart, a young doctor in his group, to take that project on.

I went to see Boshart, who is now a professor in the Biozentrum, at the Ludwig Maximilians University of Munich, on a snowy Monday morning. When I arrived at the center on the outskirts of Munich, it was virtually deserted. I could hear my footsteps echoing in the spacious hallways and supposed that the snowfall which was snarling traffic in the city was keeping people at home. But Boshart was in his office reading when I knocked on his door.

Boshart told me that he had grown up in southern Germany near Lake Constance. He had been intrigued with science from an early age and read widely—about biology, botany, biochemistry, and physics. He studied at medical schools in Munich, Montpellier, Freiburg, and Paris and was certified as a doctor. In parallel, he took science courses and became more interested in being a medical researcher than a clinician, and so he looked for a "laboratory where something was going on." He got a position in zur Hausen's lab in November of 1981, just as the research was reaching a most productive phase. The following year, when zur Hausen asked if he would look for new HPV variants in cervical cancer tumors, he gladly took on the challenge. He liked working with zur Hausen, who ran a pretty tight ship, Boshart recalled. "He came into the lab every morning. 'So,' he would ask, 'Is there something new?' Of course, we showed him something every day, because if there was nothing new . . ." Boshart frowned, imitating his mentor. "There was substantial pressure, but not in a bad way. He never said you have to provide those data in two days. But he expected that there would be productivity. He expected that we would come in early in the morning. It was totally unacceptable to be there after eight. That was the latest. There was a morning meeting every second day and if you didn't attend, you would be in a lot of trouble. He was very strict."

Boshart was ambitious and determined to succeed in the project he had been given. When he investigated one tumor of a black patient from Brazil, he could see that it contained an unusually large number of copies of a DNA sequence that was unidentified but related to papillomaviruses. Lutz Gissman, who was supervising him, said, "I think this is a very interesting tumor." But then Boshart recalled, "He wanted someone else to continue with it. Lutz was thinking he should give it to someone more experienced. I was not very happy. I went to zur Hausen and told him what I had found and that I really wanted to continue and try to isolate the sequences. He agreed to let me continue."

Boshart was under the gun to complete the project. Not only did he want to justify zur Hausen's faith in him, he also knew that he would have to leave soon to fulfill his two-year national service requirement. (In the 1980s conscription was still in full swing; it ended in 2011.) Boshart was twenty-seven and he could not postpone his duty beyond June 1982. "I had a clear deadline. I had to plan my experiments very carefully. I couldn't allow for failures. Any failures would cost me weeks. I worked very very hard. I worked until eleven in the evening most days and sometimes until midnight. The experiments were very difficult because we did so-called low-stringency hybridizations. On a background of a black image, you could see something which was a little blacker than black. This was the most advanced technique available for these questions." Determining whether one of these black-on-black images was significant required judgment, discernment. The assessment was not routine.

A couple of months after finding "the interesting tumor," Boshart knew that it contained DNA from another new member of the HPV family—eventually called 18. On his last day of work, he still had ten rolls of film to develop. He left careful instructions for his colleagues about completing this last step. Two years later, his paper describing the finding was published.[31]

Zur Hausen finally knew that 70 percent of cervical cancers contained either HPV 16 or HPV 18. These were the high-risk HPV viruses he had been seeking for so long. But convincing the rest of the scientific community still took time. At the end of July 1983, in the Swedish coastal town of Orenas, at the Second International Conference on Papilloma Viruses, Gissman and Dürst presented their findings about HPV 16. Gissman recalled, "This was not a good experience. We were really proud, Dürst and myself. We thought we had something interesting to present. Dürst spoke good English; my English was limited. There was discussion—skepticism, aggressiveness. In retrospect, you ask yourself, 'What did you do wrong?' We prepared our talks the best way we could. I did not understand many questions, what they were saying. Dürst probably understood the English better, but didn't understand the contents. It was a little bit of chaos." Zur Hausen jumped to the stage and tried to rescue the situation, but without much success. Gissman summed up the event this way: "The whole show went down the drain." Zur Hausen and his colleagues had not managed to persuade the other scientists of the significance of their findings.

Nevertheless, there were positive developments. Gissman said, "For me, a very good moment was when Peter Howley called. We had sent him the DNA very early on. He called me and said, 'I can reproduce your data. I also find it.'" Then a Czech virologist, Vladimir Vonka, published a study of ten thousand women in which he showed that the risk of developing pre-cancerous lesions in the cervix was the same for women who had antibodies to herpes as it was for those who didn't. The implication was clear: the cause lay elsewhere. The rival virus was being edged out of the running.[32]

In 1983, zur Hausen was invited to take on the position of scientific director at the DKFZ in Heidelberg. Founded in 1964, this was the largest cancer research institution in the country, but its reputation was in shambles. Newspapers were grumbling about underwhelming results and complaining that investigators were spending too much time looking at mice. Editorials muttered darkly about scientists losing sight of the fact that they were supposed to cure people. Zur Hausen had ideas about how to put the organization on a solid scientific footing and ensure that its aim—helping people—was front and center with everyone. In his years of research, he had always kept a firm grip on what it was *for*. As he explained to me, "I was not particularly interested in HPV as such." Although he spent thirty-six years studying the virus, his ultimate goal was finding the cause of cervical cancer. He said, "If the agent had turned out to be a bacterium or a parasite, it would have interested me as well."

Zur Hausen moved to Heidelberg in the spring of 1983. As he was planning to continue with his own investigations, a number of his Freiburg collaborators came with him. A year later, Ethel-Michele de Villiers also took a position there. I wrote de Villiers an email asking if I might interview her, but she politely begged off. "I appreciate the fact that you would want to interview me as well, but I hope you will understand if I decline. My 'policy' has been not to participate in these events—the prize is my husband's merit and he should enjoy everything that goes with it." When I mentioned her note to zur Hausen, he said, "I met her initially when she came to our lab from South Africa to learn some techniques. We didn't get into a personal relationship in this period. But later on, yes. [They married in 1992.] She's heading a division here in the cancer center and she would have told you, if you had spoken to her, that I am presently working as a postdoc in her laboratory." And then he laughed, clearly enjoying the idea of himself in that role again.

AN INGENIOUS IDEA

When zur Hausen started working at the DKFZ, it employed over 1,100 people, scientists and support staff, and had a budget of 85 million deutsche marks. Nevertheless, zur Hausen managed to carve out a couple of hours a day for his own research. He still had some important questions to answer. As the 1983 landmark paper about HPV 16 states: "The regular presence of HPV DNA in genital cancer biopsy samples does not *per se* prove an etiological involvement of these virus infections, although the apparent cancer specificity of HPV 16 is suggestive of such a role." HPV 16 and 18 were clearly "viruses of interest," but more evidence was required to convict. How did they cause cancer? And how could it be shown?

To hear more about that, I interviewed Elisabeth Schwarz, a biology professor at the DKFZ. When I first met her, she was striding purposefully through the halls of the institute, her lab coat flapping behind her. Schwarz exuded confidence; she struck me as someone who was entirely at home where she was. But when we sat down in a meeting room to talk, Schwarz told me that her interest in biology actually started by chance. At her high school in Wetzlar (about an hour's drive north of Frankfurt), students could choose some electives during their final year. Schwarz chose philosophy, a very popular option. It was so popular, in fact, that the class was oversubscribed. When the teacher asked if anyone might like to try biology instead, Schwarz considered the idea for a few minutes and then thought, "Okay, why not?" The class aroused her deep and abiding interest in the subject and when she entered university, she majored in it. Later she went on to do a PhD at Freiburg University, specializing in molecular biology. "The 1970s was the time when molecular biology, techniques for cloning, and DNA sequence analysis developed." For Harald zur Hausen it was, she observed, fortuitous. "With the papillomaviruses you cannot do classic virological experiments because they do not replicate in culture and so that was also a very unique and helpful combination—the hypothesis he had developed and the methodological improvements which were then available." Schwarz finished her PhD in 1979 and joined zur Hausen as a postdoc.

After Gissman and de Villiers isolated and cloned HPV 6, Schwarz began to take on the task of completely sequencing that virus. With four doctoral students in medicine and biology, she spent several months characterizing its 7,902 base pairs or nucleotides. Schwarz was a maestro of the molecular tools of the day. "Because I was engaged in DNA sequencing in my PhD work, I knew at that time the newest technology in DNA sequence analysis. I was one of the very few young scientists in Germany who could do the sequencing." (The technology has continued to improve, and now it is possible to sequence about 10 million base pairs in five days!)

Then she said, "Harald zur Hausen had an ingenious idea. He wondered whether cell lines like the famous HeLA cell line might contain human papillomavirus DNA." The "famous HeLa cell line" was derived from a cervical cancer which had killed an American black woman, Henrietta Lacks, in 1951. Her cells were the first human cells to be successfully grown in the lab; they grew very easily and prolifically. They have become the workhorse of molecular research. It is estimated that if all the HeLa cells distributed around the world were collected together today, they would weigh 800 pounds. For years, her family did not know that her "immortal" cells were being used in this way, nor that laboratories which cultured the cells were profiting by them. The story has raised complex ethical and legal issues about whether patients retain legal rights over tissues removed from their bodies. But the HeLa line continues to be used in research, and to date over sixty thousand scientific papers have been published about the cells. For more on this story, see Rebecca Skloot, *The Immortal Life of Henrietta Lacks*.[33] Cell lines remain popular with scientists because with them, it is possible to repeat an experiment many times on genetically identical cells, something which cannot be done using the alternative—cells derived from multiple tissue donors.

Zur Hausen's "ingenious idea" proved to be correct. When Schwarz looked at the HeLa cell line and two others derived from cervical cancer, she could see that all three were infected with HPV 18. Moreover, said Schwarz, "It became clear that the viral genome is not present as a circular molecule called an episome, but it seems to become part of the host cell genome. It is present in an integrated state." To show me what happened during integration, she opened a small notebook and drew the virus's original circular genome with its eight genes strung around the outside like beads. Schwarz explained that for it to fuse with the cellular genome, it had to become a linear strand—it had to open like a necklace. And, she said, this raised an important question: *Where* did the virus's circular genome open? As Schwarz drew a line through the E2 gene in her sketch, she told me that no matter which cell line she used, the break in the virus's genome always happened in the region of E2, a regulatory gene. As a result, that gene was destroyed during integration while two other viral genes, E6 and E7, were preserved in the hybrid sequence. This meant that the latter two were freed from E2's control. Since they were always present in the cancerous cells, they were candidate causal agents. Schwarz said that if E6 and E7 really were the basis of the malignancy, they would not just be present in the genome of the cancer cells, but be active as well. She set out to prove that this was so.

An active gene is one that expresses proteins, a complex process that involves ribonucleic acid or RNA, a close cousin of DNA. While DNA is normally double-stranded, RNA is usually a single strand. To create it, DNA unzips itself and one strand becomes the template for an RNA sequence. You can think of DNA as the genetic blueprint which contains all the instructions for the working of an organism. The RNA carries out those instructions and fulfills various functions in the creation of proteins. In this situation, Schwarz was interested in its role as a messenger. It copies the data held by the DNA in the nucleus of the cell and transfers it to the surrounding cytoplasm. You could say that RNA takes the genetic records from storage and delivers them to the manufacturing plant where a protein is synthesized.

Schwarz reasoned that if the cancer cells had RNA which contained instructions for making E6 and E7 proteins, this would be evidence that the corresponding genes were active. Using a radioactive probe, she detected just such a segment of RNA in the cervical cancer cells. The E6 and E7 genes were sending out messages; they were definitely active. It was more evidence that they were cancer-causing. Schwarz said, "That was the first hint that these genes are oncogenes—a result of major importance. We published in *Nature*."[34] "Sometimes the experiments failed," Schwarz said. "Nevertheless, there was steady progress." She spent eighteen months striving for publishable results, often working long hours. Zur Hausen came by every day to check on what was happening. "He realized," she recalled, "that this was the decisive period—the breakthrough time."

Then she said, "Come, I'll show you some of the original data."

I donned a white coat and followed Schwarz to the lab where her tiny office, lined with floor-to-ceiling shelves bulging with books and papers, was tucked into a corner. There was just enough room for two people to stand behind the desk which looked out over a snowy courtyard. I noticed the screensaver on her computer. It was a picture of a Norwegian ship called the *MS Kong Harald* (King Harald). I looked at Schwarz inquiringly and she laughed. She said, "I went on a cruise and that was the ship I was on. I thought it was funny."

Then Schwarz reached back onto the shelf and pulled down a binder. Leafing through it, she showed me the pictures of the laddered black bands that revealed the genetic structure of the molecules she had investigated. These were the chemical tracks of an invisible virus. "You know," she said, "it was a fantastic time. It's something that not every scientist gets to experience."

Elisabeth Schwarz's work had helped to show that the viral genes E6 and E7 were very likely the ones that initiated the carcinogenic process. Magnus von Knebel Doeberitz, a doctor who joined zur Hausen's group in Heidelberg in 1985, wondered if you could take this one step further. Could you show that these genes were also needed to *maintain* the cancer? If you knocked out those genes, would you arrest the growth of tumor cells?

I'd first heard about von Knebel Doeberitz's experiment from George Klein, who said that it was "the final convincing evidence" that showed zur Hausen's hypothesis was correct. Von Knebel Doeberitz is now head of a research group which the University of Heidelberg and the DKFZ established jointly. I met him in his office on the sixth floor of the University of Heidelberg's Institute of Pathology. As I sat down at a round table, he gestured at the window; thick fluffy snow was falling. "If it weren't for snow," he said, "you'd have a good view of the campus from here."

Von Knebel Doeberitz grew up in Hannover and Hamburg. While in high school, he was a good student, but he also enjoyed sports, mainly tennis, and a hobby, training dogs. He became interested in biology and chemistry and upon graduation entered medical school at the University of Freiburg. After hearing zur Hausen and a few of his colleagues give some lectures on virology, he joined their lab to do his medical thesis. Zur Hausen moved to Heidelberg in 1983 and von Knebel Doeberitz followed a couple of years later. For him, it was difficult to decide whether to pursue science or clinical work. He always enjoyed his interactions with patients. "I decided to stay in science because the impact of what you are doing can be substantially important for a broader range of people. That was the final decision-maker for me."

When von Knebel Doeberitz arrived in Heidelberg as a postdoc, he spun his wheels for a couple of years looking for viruses in lymphomas. He said, "This was quite frustrating. Nothing serious came out of it and hasn't to this day. That doesn't exclude that there might be viruses involved but we couldn't find them." Then he had an idea about how you could use something called anti-sense RNA to prevent oncogenes in cervical cancer cell lines from synthesizing dangerous proteins. Anti-sense RNA, discovered just a few years before, got its name from the fact that instead of transmitting a message, it blocked transmission. It bound to messenger RNA and formed a double-stranded RNA molecule. As soon as this happened, von Knebel Doeberitz told me, "it degraded rapidly within the nucleus so that the proteins encoded by those messenger RNAs couldn't be expressed—or not to the same level as they could be expressed before." Von Knebel Doeberitz spent about two years implementing his idea. In the end, it worked. E6 and E7 were true oncogenes; when their expression of proteins was blocked, tumor growth stopped. As he had suspected, they were necessary not only to initiate cancer, but also to maintain it.[35]

Von Knebel Doeberitz's results suggested that anti-sense RNA could potentially provide a way of treating patients. However, he explained, "It turned out to be extremely difficult to develop methods to block genes in human beings. You have to somehow get these anti-sense RNA sequences into their cells. That has never worked well up to now. Nobody has identified a technique where this could be applied to living organisms. But it is still an active area of research." While von Knebel Doeberitz didn't find the treatment he was hoping for, his research was, nonetheless, a significant milestone. Zur Hausen said that the work was "the final proof" that HPV caused cervical cancer, that the malignancy was unlikely to occur without it. Later it became apparent why this was so. Von Knebel Doeberitz said, "After this experiment was done, other groups, particularly Peter Howley's, investigated the biochemical action of E6 and E7." They discovered that these viral genes interfered with cellular repair mechanisms; they *de-activated* proteins that suppressed tumor growth.

A PERIOD OF FRUSTRATION

Traditionally, cancer research has aimed at finding a cure once the disease has developed. But zur Hausen's findings opened the door for a new possibility—forestalling the malignancy altogether. Fortunately, most women who contract even high-risk papilloma infections do not go on to develop cervical cancer. Co-factors probably play a role. Lifestyle choices about diet or smoking, exposure to noxious chemicals, other infections, or suppression of the immune system probably explain why some women infected with HPV progress to cancer while others do not. An HPV infection is *necessary* for cervical cancer to develop. Once it is established, the co-factors tip the balance.

The co-factors are not easy to control. But a vaccine does make it possible to prevent an HPV infection. And without the infection, the cancer will not develop—even if the "co-factors" are present. That's what makes the vaccine such an attractive option. As soon as zur Hausen had the two isolates for HPV 16 and 18, he began phoning pharmaceutical companies to see if they were interested in cooperating with him on the development of a vaccine. To his surprise, they were not enthusiastic. Only one company, Behring AG, was sufficiently impressed by zur Hausen's data to want to get on board. Then, he said, its parent company, Hoechst AG, "initiated a market analysis which came up with a totally faulty conclusion, that there would be no market." It lost interest. "That was a period of frustration for me again," he recalled. Moreover, epidemiological studies of cervical cancer and HPV viruses were confusing for awhile and discouraging to anyone who might be thinking about a vaccine. Von Knebel Doeberitz said that paradoxically, a generous impulse of zur Hausen's may also have delayed vaccine development. As soon as he had the two isolates relevant for cervical cancers, he offered them to other researchers. He wanted them to be able to confirm his results and use them for their own research. Hundreds of labs around the world took advantage of the opportunity and began working with the viral DNA. Critically, zur Hausen didn't think about getting a patent first.

Von Knebel Doeberitz recalled, "He never thought about money, about making money from science." This was true and, indeed, the attitude was typical of many German academics at the time. Later zur Hausen wrote, "Up into the 1990s, it was unpopular among most scientists at German universities and research institutes, perhaps considered even a little dishonorable, to patent scientific results. Scientists only sought to publish good results as quickly as possible."[36] In von Knebel Doeberitz's opinion, this created difficulties that zur Hausen did not foresee. He explained,

> If you look at the history of the development of the HPV vaccine, it would have gone much faster if he would have gone for a patent even in the early eighties. From my point of view it was not a mistake to make the DNA freely available. You can do that. What went wrong was not writing a patent before sending it out. Having the patent would have facilitated a lot of research that was done afterwards. You would have been able to deal with industry. Say you are the manager of a company who is thinking about supporting zur Hausen's work. You want to make a vaccine and have to invest a million dollars. You will be asked by the shareholders, "What are you doing with our money?" They need to be certain the money will benefit them as investors.

Von Knebel Doeberitz thought a lack of clarity about the ownership of rights to the discovery may have scared off some potential investors—a point most American professors would have understood but that few German academics appreciated.

Zur Hausen was blindsided in 1992 when the National Institutes of Health in the US filed a patent application for an HPV vaccine developed by two of their scientists, John Schiller and Doug Lowy. Later zur Hausen wrote, "The different attitudes with respect to patenting in the US and Germany were perhaps one of the reasons why we didn't see the American patent application coming. It incorporated part of our results without our consent. The basis of the US patent application were our DNA isolates 16 and 18, which had been sent by our laboratory to Peter Howley at the US National Cancer Institute and which he had probably passed on to Douglas Lowy and John Schiller."[37]

Five years of disheartening legal wrangling followed. Zur Hausen described them as "the wasted years." In the end, zur Hausen's employer, the DKFZ, and the National Institutes of Health in the US reached an agreement whereby the DKFZ would receive a share of future revenues from the vaccine. In 1995, the International Agency for Research on Cancer declared that HPV 16 and 18 were carcinogens,[38] and in 2006, the US Food and Drug Administration (FDA) approved Gardisil, the first HPV vaccine from Merck & Co.[39] It protected against HPV 16 and 18, the high-risk cancers responsible for 70 percent of cervical cancers, as well HPV 6 and HPV 11, the low-risk viruses which cause genital warts.

A VOICE WITH A SWEDISH ACCENT

At quarter past eleven, on the morning of October 6, 2008, Harald zur Hausen was in his office at the German Cancer Research Center in Heidelberg. He was sitting at his desk quietly editing a paper when the telephone rang.

"Zur Hausen," he answered simply, as he always did.

On the line was a voice with a Swedish accent. The man introduced himself as Hans Jörnvall, secretary of the Nobel Committee. He congratulated zur Hausen for sharing in the 2008 Prize for Physiology or Medicine. The other two laureates were Françoise Barré-Sinoussi and Luc Montagnier, who won for discovering another important virus—HIV (human immunodeficiency virus), which causes AIDS (Autoimmune Disease Syndrome). Zur Hausen was completely surprised. In 2007, he had heard rumors of being nominated for the world's most prestigious medical accolade, but nothing had come of it. Other matters quickly claimed his attention. At seventy-two, zur Hausen was busy. He held an emeritus position at the Cancer Center, was still an active researcher, and was also the editor-in-chief of the *International Journal of Cancer*. Though it was fall again "Nobel season," the possibility he might win had completely slipped zur Hausen's mind.

Jörnvall instructed z ur Hausen not to tell anyone that he had received the award until he was able to make the official public announcement. But zur Hausen could not restrain himself from making one call—to his wife, de Villiers. She was at the airport in Frankfurt, taxiing down the runway in preparation for takeoff. Fortunately, she had neglected to switch off her cell phone, and zur Hausen was able to reach her and relay the news. When a flight attendant saw that de Villiers was using a phone, she rushed over to tell her to turn it off. De Villiers said, "But my husband has just won the Nobel Prize." The flight attendant said, "Okay, then I haven't seen anything."

Lutz Gissman was in Buenos Aires, Argentina, attending some meetings about another vaccine he was developing, when he received an email with the news. "It was a big event," he said. "Even I had to give three telephone interviews. I don't know how they identified me. In the evening, I was lucky enough to reach zur Hausen." Dürst was in Jena in his lab when his wife, who had been listening to the radio, called him. "She was very, very excited," Dürst said. "Later that night, we opened a bottle of champagne and celebrated with our two daughters and our cat. I had hoped he would get the prize much earlier, but it made us very happy." Schwarz arrived in her lab late that morning. She had heard nothing while driving over, because she had been listening to music, not the radio. A colleague of hers exclaimed, "Oh Elisabeth! Have you heard? H. has won the Nobel Prize!" Shortly afterward, Schwarz said, "I will try to reach him. Then I told him how happy I was. I congratulated him."

Von Knebel Doeberitz was in Bonn in the middle of a discussion with some other German cancer experts about colorectal cancer. A colleague of his with an iPhone suddenly began winking at him in what he was sure was intended to be a meaningful way. He recalled, "I didn't understand his gesture. I had no idea the Nobel Prizes were being made public. Then he sent me an SMS, 'Your boss has got the Nobel Prize.' For everybody who was involved, this was a great event. I travelled back from Bonn, came to Heidelberg, quite late, at six or seven in the evening. I immediately went to Harald's office."

The day that was so many years in the making had finally come. "One of zur Hausen's real strengths is to think in very large and broad concepts," said von Knebel Doeberitz. "What kind of disease could be infectious although nobody knows it is? And if it is not an immanently infectious disease, what could be the reason for it? These are simple concepts—simple in the beginning, but difficult to prove in the long run. He climbed the stairway, step by step."

As zur Hausen had predicted when he was sixteen, a schoolboy in Vechta, he had won the Nobel Prize. And as he had pledged, too, he invited all of his family to join him in Stockholm to celebrate.

4

BARRY MARSHALL, ROBIN WARREN, AND *HELICOBACTER PYLORI*

We were trying to tell people that ulcers, which they knew were caused by other things, were caused by bacteria, which they knew weren't there.

—Robin Warren

A FUNNY BLUE LINE

June 11, 1979. A rainy winter day in Perth, Western Australia. It was Robin Warren's forty-second birthday, but it began like any other Monday morning. He had breakfast with his wife, Win, and his noisy brood of five children. Then he drove to the Perth Royal Hospital, where he was a pathologist. Arriving about nine o'clock, he went downstairs to the basement of the building. His office was a small, windowless room stuffed with books and papers, opposite the morgue. The air-conditioning didn't work very well, and if he was smoking one of the cigarillos in which he occasionally indulged, the air turned blue. Warren turned to his first duty—looking after the specimens that had come down to the lab during the night before. He prepared them for "sectioning" by preserving the tissues from degradation and then infusing them with a liquid, usually wax, that would solidify. This made it possible to cut very thin slices or sections of tissue that could be examined under a microscope.

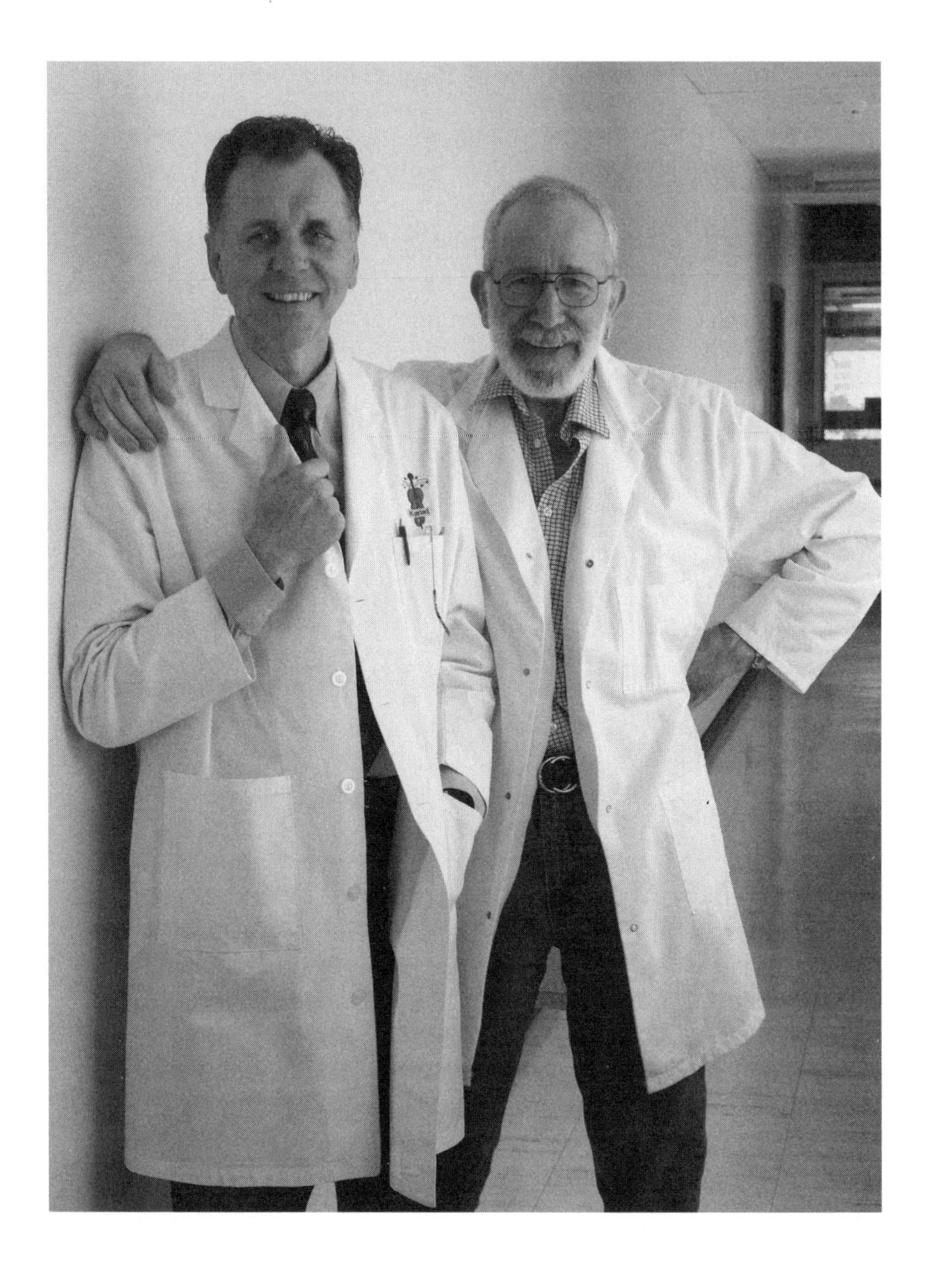

Figure 4.1. Barry Marshall and Robin Warren. Photo courtesy of Frances Andrijich

Warren had been working as a pathologist since 1962, when he started as a registrar (a specialist trainee) in Adelaide. He found the subject deeply absorbing. As he said in a 2008 interview with Norman Swan for the Australian Academy of Science, "We're always finding interesting things in pathology. When you look down the microscope at pieces of tissue, it's not unusual to find something unexpected, because there are so many unusual things. And if there are 10,000 unusual things, you find one of them every now and again."[1] For Warren, the work was never mechanical. Whenever he examined a sample, he was alive to the possibility of discovery—aware that he might be surprised.

By the afternoon of June 11, Warren had started looking at the day's new specimens. One in particular, a gastric biopsy, caught his eye. "There weren't very many of these before 1970," he told me in a long phone interview from his home in Perth, "but then the flexible endoscope came in and the gastroenterologists were taking lots of stomach biopsies." The instrument, which consisted of a tube with a light and video camera at the end, transmitted images and made it easy to take small samples of tissue. Peptic ulcers were common in those days—both gastric (in the stomach itself) and duodenal (just beyond the stomach in the first part of the small intestine). By the late seventies, Warren often processed as many as four or five gastrointestinal biopsies a day. Since stomach ulcers in particular were at risk of turning malignant, physicians wanted to be sure that the pain and discomfort of their patients was not due to cancer. The samples would usually come in with the instruction, "Peptic ulcer, query carcinoma."

Warren peered through the microscope. He could see evidence of gastritis—an inflammation of the stomach lining. For a long time, gastritis was regarded as a minor complaint, in comparison to ulcers (which erode part of the stomach lining) and cancer. But Warren had begun to pay attention to the disorder and classify it. He categorized the gastritis as "severe, chronic, and active," using a system he had adapted from Richard Whitehead, a fellow Australian.[2] Then he noticed something which he had never noticed before, something new. He said, "I just thought there was a funny blue line on the surface of the tissue. I wasn't too sure what it was and so I had a closer look with the higher power lens. It looked like a lot of bacteria were there." In his report about the biopsy, Warren wrote, "The bacteria have the morphology of *Campylobacter*."[3] These were a type of twisted or corkscrew-shaped microbe, discovered in 1963; they were one of the main causes of bacterial foodborne disease. Warren knew they often inhabited the intestines and the colon, but he was surprised to come across anything like them in the stomach.

Warren was fully aware of the standard medical teaching. He said, "Everyone thought no bacteria could grow in the stomach. It was a sort of known fact, like everyone knew the Earth was flat in the Middle Ages." Gastric acid, after all, was as corrosive as car battery acid. How would any living organism survive in it? The stomach was supposed to be the one organ in the body in which bacterial infections could not take root. (It followed from this, of course, that they did not cause stomach diseases—a point to which we will return.)

When Warren showed his singular finding to his boss, Dr. Len Matz, one of the best pathologists in Perth, he was disappointed that Matz couldn't see what he saw. Warren's three colleagues in the lab couldn't see anything unusual either. The funny blue line didn't look like bacteria to them. But Warren was sure he was right. He had a stubborn faith in the evidence of his own senses. He tried to explain his reliance on them this way: "I know you're on the phone because I'm talking to you. It is a concrete thing for me. Even if someone else doesn't believe me, I know you're there. They can tell me you're not there as much as they like. And somebody else in the room here wouldn't be able to hear you or see you. But I can hear you. So as far as I'm concerned you're there. I don't care what they say. That's what it was like."

Warren thought he could help his colleagues see the bacteria more clearly. For this he turned to a minor hobby of his—"something I did now and again for fun." Over the past ten years, he had been experimenting with the stains microbiologists and pathologists used when they were looking at tissue and wanted to highlight features of interest. He said, "Microbiologists used them on smears taken from cultures. They'd get a culture with a colony of bacteria and smear them on a glass slide so that the slide was covered with masses of bacteria. And then they'd use one of their special stains to see what sort of bacteria they were. You almost didn't need a stain; you could use pen and ink or something because there were so many of them there and there was nothing else there." Warren told me that pathologists, on the other hand, were usually looking for bacteria in human tissue—a much more complex material than a glass slide. It was harder to spot microbes there. "Even if bacteria are there, they aren't very many of them," Warren said. "And then if you want to stain the bacteria, you have to contend with the fact that both the bacteria and the tissue are living organisms. They tend to stain with the same stains. You've got to find a stain that will stain bacteria clearly and not the tissue."

Warren had tested a silver stain called Warthin-Starry on a whole range of bacteria to which it wasn't normally applied. "It seemed to work quite often," he said. "So I tried it with these [gastric] bacteria when I first saw them and it worked very nicely on them." The stain turned them dark grey while the background took on a golden-brown color. The small curved spiral organisms sticking closely to the surface of the stomach stood out clearly. "You couldn't argue with it," said Warren. He told me later in a clarifying email, "The silver stain can be difficult and it does not always work well, but when it does work well the results are excellent and beyond doubt." Warren showed the biopsy to his colleagues in the lab, and this time they agreed with him. The bacteria were there all right. "But they didn't think they were of any significance," Warren said. Matz told him, "Well look, if you think they are important, see if you can find any more."

"I didn't expect to find any more," Warren explained, "but since I was challenged, I started looking for them on all the other biopsies. Actually once you start looking for them, they are not that hard to find. They were there in about a third of the biopsies we had."

THE ONLY THING I COULD FIND WAS A JOB IN PATHOLOGY

Robin Warren is a fifth-generation Australian who was born in Adelaide in 1937. His father, Roger Warren, studied viticulture and worked for the Hardy Wine Company, one of the largest wineries in southern Australia. His mother, Helen Verco, was a nurse. She came from a family of doctors and wanted desperately to become one herself. But money was tight when she was growing up and her widowed mother, Alice, had only been able to scrape together enough money to send Helen's brother, Luke, to medical school.

When I asked Warren whether his mother had encouraged him to become a doctor, he said he wasn't sure where his attraction to medicine came from, but he allowed, "We saw a lot of my uncle who was a very nice GP, country doctor, you know. I just knew that my mom's family were doctors. She didn't try to push me into it or anything, but was always interested in it." Warren was a voracious reader as a child. He liked adventure stories for boys, books about science, even reference texts. Warren recalled, "The twelve-volume Oxford Junior Encyclopedia started to be published. It came out volume by volume. At least the first four volumes that came out, I just read them from cover to cover. After that they started coming out a bit faster and I couldn't read them that fast. I didn't read them quite cover to cover, but I looked at them all."

Warren went to St. Peter's College for his secondary education—an elite institution, the oldest school in Adelaide. Howard Florey, another Australian Nobel laureate, had studied there years before.[4] Warren described himself as a "reasonably good student." But, he said, "there was a limit to how well I fitted in, because I wasn't good at sports. At the school I went to, they expected you to be good at sports. I didn't do well from that point of view." Warren liked to go on solitary bicycling expeditions to explore the hills around Adelaide and take pictures of the scenery. He'd been fascinated by photography ever since he was a small child and watched his father taking family photos with an old Voitlander camera. He'd nagged his dad into getting him a camera, which he finally did when Warren was ten. He got a Brownie Box, then obtained developing trays and learned how to make his own prints.

In 1955, Warren entered medical school at Adelaide University. He thoroughly enjoyed all aspects of his studies—anatomy, physiology, biochemistry, pharmacology, embryology, histology. After graduating in 1961, he spent his first year as a resident at the Royal Adelaide Hospital. He bought himself a new camera, a Leica M3, and began photographing medical as well as personal subjects. While at the Royal Adelaide, Warren met Winifred Williams, who was studying obstetrics. They began spending more and more time together and married a year later. Warren described this as "the biggest and best decision of his life."[5] Their first baby was soon on the way.

Warren decided to do his second year of residency in psychiatry. "Looking back on it, I realize I was extremely naïve," he recalled.

> At the time, the Australian Medical Journal used to publish a whole section of advertisements for jobs available. What my colleagues did, what everyone did, apparently, except me, was apply for every job that they could. Then they took the one they liked best of the ones

> they were offered. What I did when I finished my intern year was apply for the job I wanted. I thought that was the polite thing to do—not to apply for every job you think you can and probably not even answer most of the ones that say yes. I just applied for the one I wanted and the short answer is that I didn't get it. Then I had to look around for something that was left over, that no one had applied for. The only thing I could find was a job in pathology.

Luckily, the work suited Warren. He'd always enjoyed sitting down with microscopes and looking at things. There was often something to learn, and he frequently found himself thinking of ways to improve how he did his work. In 1964, Warren moved to take a job as a pathologist at the Royal Melbourne Hospital. Then in 1969, he took a position at the Royal Perth Hospital. He and Win bought a house in Perth and settled in with their children (by this time, they had four sons). He stayed at the hospital in Perth until he retired thirty years later.

YOU'VE GOT TO LOOK CAREFULLY AT WHAT'S THERE

When I asked Warren why he hadn't seen the bacteria before in any of the thousands of biopsies he had examined, he said, "When you know something isn't there, it's hard to see. Our brain is not set up to see things that aren't there. There are probably things all around us that we're not seeing." And why, I asked him, did he finally notice them? Warren wasn't sure that he could explain this, but surmised that his long-standing fascination with photography might have had something to do with it. He said, "To take good photographs you've got to look carefully at what's there. When most people take a photograph, they look at the subject and snap. They don't look at what else is there. You've got to look at everything that's in front of you. That's not so easy. Usually you look at what you're interested in and forget the rest. You don't see everything. I think that probably helped me."

Warren was the right man in the right place. He had a flair for silver staining and was knowledgeable about stomach inflammation. His curiosity about the bacteria also helped, as did his contrarian streak. "I thought," said Warren, "because they weren't supposed to be there, they were particularly interesting." He had many questions about the microbes. How could they survive in the stomach when everyone knew that it was a hostile environment? Why were they there? Did they have anything to do with the inflammations he was seeing and which he had learned to classify? Noticing the bacteria was just the first step—"the easy part," as he described it in the lecture he gave when he accepted his Nobel Prize. The more difficult task was trying to understand what the microorganisms were doing in the stomach. Was there a story to tell about them? Were they more than just curiosities?

Warren found it was often surprisingly difficult to get other physicians to see the bacteria. He said, "One of the arguments they had was this: 'If the bacteria are really there, Dr. Warren, why haven't they been described before?' At that time I didn't know they *had* been described before. That was one of the main arguments against me—which just goes to show you how much anyone knew about the previous descriptions."

In fact, John Papadimitriou, an electron microscopist and a colleague of Warren's at the Royal Perth Hospital, had sighted them about a year before. Papadimitriou noticed the gastric bacteria when he was looking at a series of specimens collected by Wye Poh Fung, one of the local gastroenterologists. In a phone interview from his office in Perth, Papadimitriou recalled his observation this way:

> I looked at those biopsies and noticed the presence of these bacteria on the surface of the stomach. I thought, "That's funny." I wondered what they were and what they were doing. The question was whether we should regard them as pathogenic or commensal [living in the body without causing disease]. We thought about this for some time. We looked at those bugs and they didn't seem to penetrate the surface of the stomach. Because they didn't penetrate the gastric mucosa, we opted for the fact that they might be commensals. We didn't actually exclude that they were pathogenic and we should have. We also didn't see them in all the biopsies. We thought that they were probably not the cause, but possibly the effect of chronic gastritis. We didn't pursue the matter any further and we should have.

Thinking back, Papadimitriou said, laughing, "We made the wrong assumption." Warren had no idea that Papadimitriou had already seen the bacteria. He learned about this by accident when he visited the chief technologist in the Electron Microscopy Department at the hospital, to see if anyone there might have pictures of previous gastric biopsies.

Warren had his own pictures spread out on a table when an assistant walked by and noticed them. He said, "Hey, those are just like the ones John Papadimitriou was looking at a year or two ago." Sure enough, when Warren checked into it, he could see that the two sets of images were very similar indeed. That was when Warren learned that Papadimitriou, Fung, and Matz were authors of a three-part paper about Fung's series of biopsies.[6] When Warren got hold of it, he found that Papadimitriou mentioned finding bacteria in his section. Warren said, "He described them as something he saw, that was all." Warren is still quite puzzled by the fact that when he first noticed the bacteria and showed them to Matz, he had such a hard time seeing them. "He refused to believe that they were there even though he'd co-authored a paper that described them before. Papadimitrou described them in his part of the paper. Maybe they didn't read each other's work. I really don't know. I thought it was bizarre."

Once Warren knew about Papadimitriou's discovery, he wondered whether the microscopist might like to work with him on a paper he was planning to write about his investigations. Papadimitriou had several journal articles to his credit. Warren, who had no publications, thought it might be helpful to have someone with Papadimitriou's reputation backing him up. But Papadimitriou didn't want to get involved; at that time, he had many other projects on the go. He declined the invitation, although he encouraged Warren to continue by himself. "Keep doing your stuff, Robin, and you'll get there," he said. Papadimitriou later commented somewhat regretfully, "Ah, the twists and turns of fate."

I thought it was remarkable that these unusual bacteria, which thousands of pathologists around the world were apparently *not* seeing, had been spotted in one hospital twice in close succession. I asked both Warren and Papadimitriou if there was a reason for this. Was there something about the intellectual climate in Perth—or in the hospital? Warren said, "It's just pure chance that two people in the same department saw the things." Papadimitriou agreed: " It was a coincidence."

Even when other physicians conceded that Warren had found bacteria in some of the stomach biopsies, they rarely recognized their potential significance. Warren said, "The best I could get was, 'If they are there, Dr. Warren, they are probably secondary to the inflammation.' It was hard to prove that they *weren't* secondary to the inflammation. I didn't think they were, because they didn't *look* like it. But when someone argues like that it's difficult to prove it one way or another." For two years, Warren struggled on alone. Papadimitriou recalled, "He sat for hours and hours and hours looking down a microscope, looking at these tiny biopsies, making sure that he was seeing bacteria and making sure that they were also present in people's chronic gastritis. We're talking about close to a year of hard work, maybe more. He was very focused, very precise, very careful. I think that's what made the observations worthwhile. He has that sort of mind, that sort of attitude, that sort of focus on everything he does." Warren wrote, "In fact, there was only one doctor who did believe in what I was doing; my wife, Win, who was a psychiatrist, and who encouraged me."[7]

Methodically, Warren began assembling a series of cases. He was seeing bacteria on a regular basis. He had also noticed that they were associated with a kind of inflammation that Richard Whitehead, his reference on this subject, described as an "active change." It made the stomach take on a cobblestone look instead of appearing flat. Warren explained, "This is an unusual sort of change in the gastric epithelium, the surface layer of the stomach, which tended to occur in some cases of gastritis. I found that the cases that were infected seemed to have this active change. I'd seen the active change before, many times, but I hadn't realized that patients with this active change had this infection. That's the only thing I found that seemed to be closely related. If you ever saw the active change you could always find the bacteria."

Warren told me he was handicapped in his investigations because of his role as a pathologist. Understandably, the gastroenterologists usually sent him biopsies from visible lesions such as ulcers. This is what they needed to help them treat their patients. But these samples weren't geared toward Warren's research purposes. Ulcers often inflamed the tissue around them, so it was difficult to show exactly what effects the bacteria might be causing. For that, Warren needed to look at bacteria and tissue that was not near an ulcer—something he rarely saw in the normal course of events. Warren also didn't know much about the patients whose stomach biopsies he was examining, which also made it difficult to form a complete picture of what was happening. Nevertheless, he carried on. By July 1981, Warren thought he probably had just about enough material for a publication. Then one afternoon, fate intervened. A lanky young man by the name of Barry Marshall knocked at his door.

LIVING DANGEROUSLY

Barry Marshall was born in 1951 in Kalgoorlie, Western Australia, a rough-and-ready mining town of about 8,500 people, located 375 miles east of Perth. The red dusty land is classic outback country, studded with gum trees, dry and hot most of the year. The town's name comes from an aboriginal word meaning "silky pear," but its most famous product is gold—much of it found in The Golden Mile, a tract of land known for having the richest deposits on earth. Marshall was the eldest of four children. His mother, Marjorie, was a nurse and his father, Bob, a machinist. Kalgoorlie, Marshall said in an early-morning phone interview from his home in Perth, formed him as someone who liked to "live dangerously":

> In those days you found your own amusements. Everyone had bigger families. There would always be half a dozen children running around in the streets. I probably had a 300- to 400-meter radius around my house. There were children all different ages, backgrounds, mixing together, roaming around, doing things after school hours. There was a lot of dangerous stuff around in Kalgoorlie. You could buy fireworks and I'm sure there were guns around. If you wanted to get some gold, you could get that too. A couple of times, when my cousin and I were nine or ten years old, we walked out of town until we found a gold mine, a defunct gold mine. There were holes in the ground, like in Colorado, and you could find some rocks and chip away at them. Obviously, you wouldn't want your kids walking around these days near 200-foot-deep mine shafts.
>
> Later when we moved to Perth, I was very interested in science and chemistry. The great thing about chemistry was that you could make explosives out of fireworks. I was pretty interested in that—though not very well versed in the safety aspects. We burned our eyebrows off a few times. Luckily we still have all our fingers. We were always melting things. I remember one year we made a blast furnace in our backyard and were melting glass. Pretty good for ten-year-olds.

Marshall's mother coached him in academics. She encouraged him to read and to visit the library. Marshall said, "As a kid, I used to read biographies. I read Thomas Edison's biography, when I was around ten years old. I took it out of the library. I thought it was incredibly exciting to invent the Morse code or the lightbulb. I had this feeling that I would like to do something that Thomas Edison used to do—invent stuff." Marshall also read his mother's medical and nursing books, which gave him some understanding of anatomy and physiology. From an early age, he was interested in medicine. "I wasn't just at the receiving end," he said. If he was given a shot, he'd ask, "This needle I'm getting, what's that's for, how does that work?" And when somebody in Kalgoorlie who went to university was accepted into medical school, Marshall still recalls that it made an impression on him. "I can't remember who that was, someone who was ten years older than me, but it was a terrific thing for people in Kalgoorlie, that there was a kid there who got into medical school in Perth. The fact that I somehow knew about that makes me think it must have been discussed. I thought, 'Wow, medical school.' The seeds were there."

Marshall said, "Father had several tickets—for refrigeration, for Caterpillar marine diesel engines. So he had half a dozen technical books about electricity, physics, mechanics. Refrigeration was actually quite involved with concepts like entropy that were hard to understand." Marshall often used the resources of his father's shop to build or fix things. "I was always encouraged to take things apart. The sad thing is I couldn't always get them back together. I had trouble from time to time with my grandmother's clock. It would be back together and there would be some extra pieces sitting there on the table." Marshall said that he also had a Newnes' Children's Encyclopedia, a treasure trove of information about ideas and activities. He explained, "There are books now with chapters extracted from these old encyclopedias that were done in England in the thirties. I have one here that someone gave me—*The Dangerous Book for Boys*, the Australian edition. You could go to those little experimental chapters, things you can do. The boys would learn how to make gunpowder or rockets. Tinkering with gadgets "still amuses me," said Marshall. "If my cell phone breaks, I could go out and get a new cell phone for $300 or I could spend a whole weekend pulling it to bits and finding a little broken thing and soldering it back on. I'd be much happier doing that—wasting the whole weekend."

In his last year of high school, Marshall narrowed his career choices down to two—a doctor or an electrical engineer. In the end, he opted for medicine. He thought his math skills weren't strong enough for engineering and besides, he wasn't keen on calculus. He liked the idea of doing anatomy and physiology and understanding the human body. In 1968, he entered the University of Western Australia. He had no great ambitions beyond becoming a medical doctor. "At first, I thought everything was discovered and then I realized that there were millions of things that weren't properly understood. There were a lot of things you couldn't treat properly. I wasn't happy anymore just to be a GP treating patients on a formula." Marshall decided to become a specialist to be able to help "the one patient out of twenty that's a bit different, that's difficult. If you put me into general practice you'd go broke. Every time someone walked in without a proper diagnosis, I'd say, 'Let's do every investigation known to man.'"

While still a student, Marshall met an attractive psychology major, Adrienne. They married in 1972 ,and Luke, the first of their children, was born in 1973. Three daughters followed: Bronwyn in 1975, Caroline in 1978, and Jessica in 1981. Marshall began his specialist training in 1978 at the Queen Elizabeth II Medical Centre and a year later moved over to the Royal Perth Hospital because he wanted to become more familiar with cardiology and open heart surgery.

Marshall was interested in many aspects of clinical medicine—geriatrics, oncology, rheumatology. He also had a "can-do" attitude that was somewhat unusual among medical students. As he observed in another interview: "We'd be measuring the blood pressure on a frog, or connecting up electric volts and making a frog leg twitch, for example. Typically, a lot of the medical students came from professional families, with dads who were lawyers or doctors or professors, and they'd never ever had a chance to play around with an electrical device or tubes or pipes and pressure and things like that. I felt that I was in demand, and straight away I could see that I was able to get things going."[8] As far as he was concerned, he told me, "Nothing physical was too difficult. It was just a matter of finding the right book that would tell you how to do it. Once you understand the working of the human body, you realize it's like plumbing. It's a bunch of pipes connected to a pump, and lots of different parts will malfunction and you've got to find the blockage or narrowing and fix that." For Marshall, the 1970s and 1980s were an exciting time to be starting in medicine. More and more, doctors were relying on machines to tell them how their patients were doing. Unlike some people "who get a bit spooked by technology," Marshall was always comfortable with it. "I grew up thinking everything is a black box with something going on inside it."

In July 1981, Barry Marshall was starting his term as the new medical registrar for gastroenterology. He had asked his boss, Dr. Tom Waters, the head of the gastroenterology division, whether there was a research project he could undertake. Waters did, in fact, have a suggestion—a statistical analysis. The division had been accumulating reports on its endoscopy results and storing the information on punched cards. There was one card for each patient, and notches indicated which condition affected an individual—one for a duodenal ulcer, another for a gastric ulcer, and so on. Before the advent of personal computers, this system was a way of "crunching numbers." Marshall looked at the two-foot stack of twenty thousand cards. The idea of going through them all was daunting, and tabulating the prevalence of various endoscopy results didn't seem all that interesting. When he expressed reluctance about the project, Waters suggested he see Dr. Warren. He told Marshall that Warren had been seeing bacteria in the stomach biopsies of some patients and that he was looking for a clinical collaborator to follow up on these findings. Waters handed him a list of people afflicted by the unusual condition Warren had observed. Recalling this, Warren told me, "I think he was being a little sarcastic, actually, 'Oh, if you don't like the subject we've got, go and see what Dr. Warren's doing.'"

Marshall glanced down the list and recognized the name of a woman he had seen the term before during his internal medicine rotation. She had complained of chronic abdominal pain, but her endoscopy indicated no ulcer. Marshall was dismayed when he learned that her senior physician had referred her to a psychiatrist. "She struck me," Marshall said, "as intelligent and articulate—not the least bit mad." The case piqued his interest. He wondered whether bacteria could be responsible for the woman's problems. He decided to go downstairs and see Warren.

As Marshall sat down to look at slides of stomach biopsies, he was expecting to hear about a project that involved a few months of research. He thought that if he was lucky, he might net an interesting paper published in an obscure medical journal. He had no idea where knocking on Warren's door would lead.

I'D GET TO PROVE EVERYONE WRONG

Initially, Warren and Marshall spent a couple of hours together. Warren said, "He wasn't really all that impressed. Anyway, he didn't know what I was showing him. I think it was the first time he sat down with a microscope. I showed him the stuff I was looking at—the bacteria, the inflammation they were related to, the cases. I told him I didn't know if the bacteria were related to anything else—just the inflammation, as far as I was concerned. That's what I saw, you see—a little piece of tissue with some inflammation and some bacteria. That's all I had for each case. I didn't know what else the patient had. That's where Barry could come in." Warren explained to Marshall that he needed biopsies of apparently normal tissue from areas of the stomach nowhere near an ulcer—that these would show the changes, the bacteria, and the inflammation better. Marshall agreed to send Warren what he needed.

Though Warren thought Marshall wasn't all that impressed, he was probably more enthusiastic than his manner let on. Marshall wrote about Warren, "He did know an awful lot about gastric histology, but after a few hours in his office, I felt my brain was full."[9] Marshall was thirty, and most of what Warren was telling him was new. As he had just started as a gastroenterology registrar, he wasn't invested in a particular theory or approach. But the idea that there might be bacteria in the stomach didn't strike him as outlandish at all. He told me he was aware that in the mid-sixties bacteria were discovered in the geysers in Yellowstone Park.[10] They survived comfortably in temperatures which up until then were considered lethal to any organism. If bacteria could thrive in liquid that was sometimes hotter than boiling water, it wasn't much of a stretch to think that some might also have evolved ways of dealing with corrosive acid. Marshall was persuaded by Warren that his microbes were probably linked to disease. However, he thought that even if this could not be shown, the discovery of a new bacterium could in itself be the subject of a publication—a welcome possibility for a young doctor wanting to make a name for himself. He had seen how much interest the newly found *Campylobacter* aroused; these gastric microbes could very well be just as intriguing.

I asked Warren what it was like to work with Marshall. He said, "He was a pretty wild young man. He gradually settled down. He was very impatient, very pushy. I don't think he was careful enough really. He wanted to get everything done. Get it done, get it done, get it out, this sort of thing. I was the person who sat down in the laboratory; he was the entrepreneur who told everybody about it. But we complemented each other—very well, in fact." Marshall echoed this assessment: "Apart from the obvious conflict between my attention deficit disorder and his obsessional perfectionism, we got on well."[11] Marshall was outgoing, sometimes described as "brash." Warren, who was sixteen years older, was more introverted. He was diligent and fastidious. He tended to worry about whether he'd gotten an observation absolutely correct, and would check and recheck his data. But there was one quality which the two men shared: they were both iconoclasts. As I mentioned, Warren said he was particularly interested in the bacteria "*because they weren't supposed to be there.*" And Marshall told me that he was excited by Warren's research because if it worked out, it meant, "*I'd get to prove everyone else wrong.*"

AN ABSOLUTE BLACK AND WHITE DIFFERENCE

Marshall left the office with Warren's favorite reference, Whitehead's description of gastritis, tucked under his arm. He started immersing himself in the study of gastric disease and curved gastric bacteria. He recalled:

> The literature was very isolated. It was not like you could find it in a literature search. In those days, books were much more important. Somebody who knew the field would write a chapter and put the key references in it. The way you found things was to go to the book chapter and then follow those references. We tracked *Helicobacter* back a hundred years. Robin and I argued about whether he discovered it or I did, but probably he did: there was a pathology encyclopedia of gastroenterology in five different volumes—dated to the mid-sixties. In it was a big picture of a *Helicobacter* taken by a professor at Harvard—Ito.

Susummu Ito was an American cell biologist, born in 1919. During World War II, he served in the all Japanese-American 442 Regiment, famous for its role in relieving the so-called Lost Battalion, a unit which the Germans had surrounded. Although the unit suffered many fatalities, Ito was unscathed in the fighting. When he returned to the United States, he went to university on the GI Bill and earned a PhD in biology. Eventually he became a professor of anatomy at Harvard and devoted himself to studying the stomach. He wrote, "I became fascinated by its unusual cells and the mysteries of its unique secretory functions."[12] An early user of the electron microscope, Ito studied cats' stomachs and took pictures of the corkscrew-shaped bacteria he found there. He was so interested in the swimming ability of these microorganisms that he made a 16 mm movie about them and showed it at a meeting of the American Society for Cell Biology. In the encyclopedia entry Ito had written, Marshall found references to a young American doctor, Stone Freedberg, who was working in Boston in 1939. Freedberg had examined thirty-five stomach specimens obtained from patients with peptic ulcers or stomach cancer and found bacteria in 40 percent of them.[13] Other researchers failed to confirm his results, however, and attributed his findings to "contamination." Marshall said, "Freedberg put his tail between his legs and said, 'I can't compete with this. I must be mental or something.' He went off and became a famous cardiologist." Fifteen years later, Dr. Eddy Palmer, a distinguished physician whose patients included President Dwight Eisenhower, also looked for the bacteria. While head of gastroenterology at Walter Reed Army Medical Center in Washington, Palmer launched a major research project to find them.[14] Marshall recounted:

> In those days, if you were the top professor at Walter Reed, you were close to God. He [Palmer] and his research fellows did a study on 1,000 people, a massive number, and could not see the bacteria in a single one. That paper that came out of Walter Reed in the fifties that said there weren't bacteria was 180 degrees in the wrong direction. The only thing you could say was that this fellow, Palmer, was so overbearing that if his research fellows missed a deadline, they would just make up the data. They found out what he thought and gave him the result that fulfilled the hypothesis that he had. Everybody who has looked at that paper says they did not do the research. They made it up. You could not look at hundreds of people without finding *Helicobacter*. They were specifically looking for it and they said, "It's not there."

Soon Marshall had found half a dozen researchers who had found spiral bacteria in the stomach and studied them different ways. The earliest reference was to an Italian pathologist, Giulio Bizzozero, who had seen them in the stomachs of dogs in 1892.[15] Marshall said, "It was reassuring that if people were observant and did a proper experiment where they documented what they saw, they would see the bacteria. It showed that it wasn't some strange bug that lived in Perth. We had international literature."

Marshall could hardly wait to put his new knowledge to the test. If, as Warren suspected, the bacteria caused stomach inflammation, it wasn't a great extrapolation to think that they might cause ulcers too. Then antibiotics could be used to treat patients—a radical departure from conventional thinking. Doctors knew that some ulcers were triggered by anti-inflammatory drugs such as aspirin and ibuprofen. However, they thought that most were psychological in origin. They had the idea that if you were under stress, or fretted or worried a great deal, your stomach responded by producing excess acid. Eating spicy foods, drinking alcohol, and smoking exacerbated the situation. In the sixties, physicians had very little to offer ulcer patients. They counseled them to live moderately and avoid excitement. An encyclopedia entry of the day captures the spirit of the advice: "It is, however, best to avoid spices, gas-forming foods and alcohol or other irritants. Since coffee, chewing gum and tobacco stimulate gastric secretions, their use should also be discontinued if possible. In addition, a person with an ulcer should understand the nature of the disease so that he may reorient himself to a life of moderation, relieve nervousness and anxiety and obtain adequate rest and sleep." If this failed they provided surgery. As the encyclopedia continued quite coolly, "Surgical treatment may be necessary in approximately 10% of all cases . . . the ulcer is removed along with three-fourths of the stomach."[16] The remedy, removing part or all of the stomach, was drastic. But it was occasionally necessary, since if an ulcer perforated the wall of the stomach, the condition was life-threatening. Without treatment, a small but significant number of patients died. But by the mid-seventies, a couple of drugs, Zantac and Tagamet, ushered in a new era for ulcer patients—and for the drug companies. These pharmaceuticals were called H2 blockers because they inhibited a chemical called Histamine2 which signaled the stomach to produce more acid. They were far better at healing ulcers than anything else that had so far been tried. Since ulcers were widespread (one in ten Americans would develop one at some time in their lives), prescriptions for the new treatments skyrocketed. The problem with the drugs, though, was that patients often had to take them indefinitely to prevent a relapse. Marshall hoped that if you could find the right antibiotic, you might be able to eradicate the bacteria in a few weeks and actually cure people—a much more satisfactory solution.

A few months after Marshall and Warren started working together they decided to test this idea of using an antibiotic and give a patient tetracycline. Marshall recalled:

> He was cured, this guy who had been driving every doctor crazy for years with his abdominal pain. He was an old fellow, a Russian guy, about eighty. For twenty years he had suffered from this pain and all of a sudden he was better. We were pretty blown away by that. When you'd see him on your list of outpatients, you'd think, "Oh my God, that guy is so depressing, we can't figure out what's wrong with him." He walked in and he was better, singing our praises. "Doctor, this treatment is fabulous." This had never happened. Antibiotics was the only thing that you had up your sleeve in medicine, that would cure people and make them miraculously better. I suppose it was like the discovery of penicillin in the forties. The doctors who were doing that were totally driven, it was so dramatic.

Though the patient was ecstatic with the results, not much could be concluded from one case. Marshall and Warren could not prove the crux of the matter—that the gastric bacteria Warren had discovered were pathogens. They decided that a proper study was needed and concluded that one which investigated one hundred patients was feasible with the limited resources they had. Marshall would finish his stint in gastroenterology at the end of 1981, and then in early 1982 move on to hematology. During the second half of that year, he was slated to work in a hospital at Port Hedland, a small mining town over 1,200 miles north of Perth. These were complications, but not insurmountable ones.

Marshall designed a protocol for the gastroenterologists and microbiologists at Royal Perth Hospital to carry out, and Stewart Goodwin, head of the Microbiology Department, gave him permission to do the research. Marshall's idea was to ask patients who were to have an endoscopy whether they would like to participate in a study. If they agreed, two biopsies would be taken. Warren would take one to correlate the presence of bacteria with gastric pathology—inflammation or peptic ulcers. Microbiologists would use the other to look for bacteria and see if they could be cultured. Marshall needed the culture in order to fulfill Koch's postulates that specified when an organism caused a disease. One of these required taking microbes grown in pure culture and using them to induce a disease experimentally—usually in an animal. While Marshall had never cultured bacteria before, he was, typically, quite confident he could do it. As he said in an earlier interview: "Although there was a lot of hocus-pocus—'It's all very difficult and you have to have your microbiology license,' et cetera—I was never fazed by that. I felt there was nothing out there that I couldn't do, if I had a go at it and learned enough about it."[17]

The research started while Marshall was working as a hematology registrar. To culture the bacteria, Marshall suggested a method developed by Adrian Lee, a microbiologist at the University of New South Wales in Sydney. He had been able to grow curved bacilli by putting them on a nutritious medium and keeping them in a low-oxygen atmosphere. Since Marshall thought the bacteria he wanted to culture looked a lot like the ones Lee had been studying, he expected they could be grown with a similar technique. But for months, the lab in the Perth Hospital had no success whatsoever. Marshall recalled:

> We had been culturing them in different ways for six months and having no luck for various reasons. Because there was limited capacity in the microbiology department, they had put our specimens into the feces culture lab. In feces, things grow like crazy and it's very contaminated, so if it hasn't grown in two days, the culture is covered in mold and all kinds of things by then. They throw it in the bin.

But on the Easter weekend, by chance, the normal procedure was not followed. The lab was short-staffed and a *Staphylococcus aureus* outbreak in one of the hospital wards meant that hundreds of employees had to be screened for an infection. The lab technicians were so busy that the gastric bacteria were neglected. Marshall said:

> Out of 100 patients, it was patient 37, I think. The week after Easter, I ran down to the lab at 2:30, 3:00 in the afternoon. The head of

> micro, John Pearman, showed it to me. He was all smiles. He was smart enough to identify that there was something new. The only reason that it showed up was that it was biopsied on Thursday and they didn't look at it until Tuesday, five days later. Nearly all *Helicobacters* will grow in five days. It wasn't totally contaminated. The idea of throwing them out after two days was a strategy you used in the feces lab, but obviously they needed to leave it a little bit longer. I looked under the microscope. I said, "These bacteria don't look like the ones in the stomach. Are you sure? Do it again and then I'll believe you." So two weeks later, he had three more cases. I then started to get a bit more interested. I said, "Great! Now we can see what antibiotics to use. We can try to infect animals to see if they get ulcers."

By May 1982, the data on a hundred patients was collected. Marshall headed off to the hospital in Port Hedland with his wife, Adrienne, and his four children. On weekends, and late into the night, Marshall collated and organized the information he had on the endoscopy patients. Then he mailed it to a statistician at Perth Royal Hospital, who sent the results back to him in September. They were compelling. Marshall said, "There was this absolute black and white difference between the biopsies if they had the bacteria or if they didn't. With bacteria you had the white blood cells. If there were no bacteria, there were no white cells either. It was like night and day. It was an amazing association. The only way you could get white cells was if you had the bacteria. There was nothing else that did it." In total, fifty-eight of the study participants had the bacteria. Almost everyone with active chronic gastritis was infected. A hundred percent (thirteen out of thirteen) of patients with duodenal ulcers had the microbes. Of the twenty-two patients with gastric ulcers, eighteen were infected. The four exceptions were people taking nonsteroidal anti-inflammatory drugs.[18] The association between bacteria and inflammation that Warren had noticed was confirmed. A picture in which the inflammation seemed to be a precursor to more serious conditions was beginning to emerge.

Marshall expected that the results would impress the medical community as much as they did him. But he was mistaken. "Coming up through medical school and reading scientific papers in training and medicine, I had the false impression that if you had statistical proof of something, people would believe it. Not necessarily so. If it is compatible with what they already know and this is an extrapolation, they're like, 'Good, we've moved on.' But they had totally different ideas about ulcers, they couldn't really take it to heart, assimilate that information. I had the wrong idea about statistics. To turn around someone's current beliefs, you've got to have a good explanation, plus all the other bells and whistles. Then people will accept the statistics."

PLUS ALL THE OTHER BELLS AND WHISTLES

In October 1982, Marshall presented the findings from his study to the local College of Physicians and Surgeons. It received "a patronizing and mostly negative response."[19] Undeterred, he and Warren decided to write a paper for the distinguished journal *Lancet*. But it was slow going. Warren said, "I was insisting that it all be correct and so on and Barry wanted it to be faster." Marshall wanted it to be clear who had described the bacteria first and so he suggested that Warren write something less ambitious that he could get out quickly—a letter. Warren said, "I thought that sounded sensible." In the end, the men wrote two letters. Warren wrote one describing the work he had done before he met Marshall, and Marshall wrote another that described the work they did together. First the letters had to appear, and that alone would take months.

In January 1983, Marshall left Port Hedland and took a position as senior registrar in gastroenterology at Fremantle Hospital, about ten miles south of Perth. This was the smallest teaching hospital in the Perth area, but it had a new research laboratory and an excellent microbiology department. His supervisor, Ian Hislop, and other colleagues there were congenial and receptive to his ideas. Marshall repeated the experiments he had done earlier, and the results were confirmed, thus proving the findings were not an idiosyncratic outcome pertaining just to the patients of Royal Perth Hospital. In February, Warren and Marshall wrote an abstract for submission to a meeting of the Gastroenterological Society of Australia. Because the meeting was local, it would not cost a great deal for them to attend and present a paper, which appealed to them. And they were sure it would be accepted. But the work was rejected. Marshall said, "It didn't even have a poster. If you don't get a poster, it's like you were faking it." [Marshall was particularly galled by this because at medical conferences, posters are of less importance than papers. The standards for them are lower. Often as many as can fit will be accepted. That the organizers of the Gastroenterological Society's meeting did not allow him to submit a poster meant they thought his work was clearly beyond the pale.] The letter Marshall and Warren received about their research just rubbed salt into the wound. It explained that sixty-seven papers were submitted but only fifty-six could be accepted. "Thus our material must have been rated in the bottom 10%!" Marshall wrote.[20]

One of Marshall's colleagues, David McGechie, a microbiologist, thought that members of his profession might be more receptive to his ideas than physicians were. He gave Marshall the phone number for Martin Skirrow, a *Campylobacter* expert who worked at the Worcester Royal Infirmary in England. By then, Marshall was coming to believe that the gastric bacteria were similar to *Campylobacter* in many ways, though probably a new species. Like *Campylobacter*, they were curved, and they could be cultivated using similar methods. But there were differences too. *Campylobacter* had one flagellum, a hair-like filament that whipped back and forth, giving the microbe motility. The gastric microorganisms had up to five sheathed flagella—a significant distinction. And of course, the fact that these bacteria could apparently live drenched in acid made them especially intriguing.

Marshall called Martin Skirrow, and it turned out that McGechie was right. Skirrow *was* interested. Skirrow is now an honorary emeritus consultant microbiologist with the United Kingdom Health Protection Agency. When I called him up at his home in England, Skirrow remembered:

> Early in 1983 the phone rang in my office one morning, and a voice said, "Hi, I'm Barry Marshall." He described this organism which looked *Campylobacter*-like and asked me whether I would like to look at it. I told him I would see what I could do with it. I told him we would be more than pleased to have it. I thought it was unique. We had never seen an organism in myriads on the lining of the stomach. It was quite new. To a microbiologist it was absolutely fascinating. I also suggested that he include his organism at a *Campylobacter* workshop to be held later in the year. It was easy for me to get it accepted. I had no idea they were having such difficulty in Australia. I didn't know either that they were having difficulty with

> the *Lancet* even. At one point David Sharp, a chap I knew on the *Lancet* editorial board, phoned me and asked, "What do you make of this?" I said I thought it was great stuff. That might have helped [them] get their first publication.
>
> At the time, Barry was just a registrar, but he would address senior colleagues, gastroenterologists, physicians, and so on, and tell them quite bluntly that they got it all wrong, that ulcers were an infectious disease. It went down like a lead balloon. They didn't realize what a brilliant man he was. He really knew his stuff on the broader issues. He was quoting Osler on acute gastritis. It wasn't a recognized syndrome in modern times. He'd dug out this work of Osler, who gave a classical description of hypochlorhydric gastritis. That was right at the beginning. He was a very bright young man who read broadly. [Later, in a clarifying email, Skirrow explained that hypochlorhydric gastritis was a low concentration of acid in the stomach that often resulted from a first infection with *H. pylori.*]

As we saw, Warren had *rediscovered* the bacteria. Over the past hundred years, other investigators had spotted them several times before. However, for various reasons, after being recognized for a brief period, the microbes had always slipped into oblivion. Another key aspect of Marshall's research was also a rediscovery—finding that bismuth could be used to treat stomach pain and disorders. A heavy metal, bismuth is a chemical cousin to arsenic and antimony, but less toxic. Bismuth subsalicylate is the active ingredient in Pepto-Bismol, the familiar, pink liquid used as an over-the-counter remedy for stomach and intestinal upset. Marshall explained:

> Bismuth is something that people have been taking for two hundred years. The middle-aged woman I was telling you about with the abdominal pain would have received bismuth subnitrate, if she had lived in Germany. They still had it on the market in Germany. Unfortunately, Australia tended to follow the US and British evidence base. The concept [in the US and Britain] was that bismuth was an anti-acid. In about 1950, a group in California that had an ulcer research establishment at UCLA wanted to know what the best anti-acid was. They said, "Let's get all the anti-acids and test them all. We won't be using the weak ones; we'll use the strong ones and fix up all the ulcer patients." They did that and the bismuth was at the low end of the scale as being an anti-acid. They said, "It's a waste of time

> using that. Let's put more aluminium and Maalox-type compounds in and less bismuth. Let's get rid of it, it's pretty useless." They changed their anti-acid, took the bismuth out. In the US after the 1940s, bismuth disappeared. Nobody had it in their medicine anymore. In Europe, the Germans said, "We've been using bismuth for two hundred years; we don't like the idea of chucking it out." They kept their anti-acid with bismuth in it. They had nothing in the US for *Helicobacter* except Pepto-Bismol, which was snake oil as far as most people were concerned. It was in the supermarket, so not a proper medicine. Procter & Gamble had bought the company. They were scratching their heads, thinking, "It's just snake oil, but we're selling $200 million a year and some people swear by it." I looked around the world at different ulcer treatments and I noticed there was an ulcer treatment with bismuth in it, called DeNol. There were reports that it cured some people with ulcers. The recurrence rate for ulcers was almost 100 percent. But if you took this treatment, the recurrence rate was 60 percent. About 40 percent of people had been cured by taking this treatment for two months. The only way I could explain this was that the stuff was actually an antibiotic. I looked in the literature and before penicillin, sure enough, bismuth used to be used for all kinds of things. It was used to treat syphilis, another curvy bacterium, a bit like *Helicobacter*.

In late April of 1983, Marshall decided to test the anti-microbial properties of DeNol. He dosed some bacteria with it and left the mixture in an incubator over a weekend. On the Monday morning when he returned to the lab and opened up the incubator, he could hardly contain his excitement. It was clear that the bismuth was inhibiting the growth of the bacteria. In vitro, they were "exquisitely sensitive" to the bismuth compound. Later, Marshall subjected the anti-acids conventionally used in the treatment of ulcers to the same test, but they had no effect on the bacteria. This explained the reports Marshall had seen—why patients taking DeNol were less likely to suffer a relapse than if they took anti-acid pills. The DeNol had an antibiotic effect, whereas the conventional drugs did not. Marshall recalled:

> People ask if I had a eureka moment. Well, that was the eureka moment. That proved that from our hypothesis, you could end up with this experiment: "Bismuth must kill *Helicobacter*." You do that experiment, and sure enough it does. That tells you your hypothesis

> is good—strong. From there you can make these quantum leaps in different directions, predict what's going to happen. All of sudden, the diverse facts that you've got in every different direction, you can extrapolate out from the *Helicobacter*. You could see some kind of article from the literature in 1950 and you could look at it and say, "I know why that happened." You could go to the paper and search through it, and sure enough, find *Helicobacter*. Even before we did our human studies, we knew we were correct.

In June 1983, Marshall and Warren's letters to the *Lancet* about "unidentified curved bacilli" were finally published. Marshall concluded his piece by succinctly staking out the intellectual territory. "If these bacteria are truly associated with antral gastritis [inflammation of the lower part of the stomach], as described by Warren, they may have a part to play in other poorly understood, gastric associated diseases (i.e., peptic ulcer and gastric cancer)."[21] These bacteria, he was telling the world, might have a role not only in gastritis and ulcers, but also in cancer. His two sentences presaged a revolution. But it would take time to unfold. When I asked him how people reacted, he said, "The letters got virtually no reception. There were a few microbiologists who read them. But gastroenterologists could not assimilate it or use it. They would hardly ever treat anybody with antibiotics. Infectious disease was not what they did."

Fortunately, Marshall and Warren did get another chance to reach an international audience. Thanks to Martin Skirrow's enthusiasm, they were invited to speak at the workshop in Brussels. At this three-day conference on the campus of the French university in Brussels, Université libre de Bruxelles, many participants gave oral and poster presentations—152 in all. But in his opening remarks, Skirrow singled out Warren and Marshall's talk for special mention. He reported that just before coming to Brussels, Marshall had visited a clinic in England and had found the bacteria in a woman with a gastric ulcer. Skirrow pointed out, "So the bacteria are not exclusively Australian." In other words, they were not a microscopic equivalent of Australia's exotic macroscopic fauna—kangaroos, wallabies, koalas, and the like. Skirrow said that there was a "burning question": were these organisms the primary or the secondary causes of peptic ulcers? "That high priority should be given to finding an answer goes without saying," he said.[22] The first slide that Marshall put up was of *Australia II*, the upstart yacht from

Perth that was going to challenge the *US Liberty* in the 1983 America's Cup. Skirrow said to me, "That was typical Barry Marshall. He rubbed it in." (The Australian boat would win, breaking the 132-year American winning streak.) Despite the glowing introduction, not everyone in the audience was convinced. One of the skeptics was Dr. Martin Blaser, an American doctor who had been studying *Campylobacter* at his lab in Colorado. Marshall recalled, "After I'd presented this data, he stood up and said, 'Dr Marshall, you're saying that some cases of peptic ulcer are caused by these bacteria?' I said, 'Not exactly. I'm saying that *all* cases of peptic ulcer are caused by these bacteria.' *Some cases* was a big leap as far as he was concerned." Later Blaser told Terence Monmaney, who was writing an article about Marshall, that at the time, his talk struck him as "the most preposterous thing I'd ever heard." He thought, "This guy is a madman."[23]

But more microbiologists started to get excited by the bacteria. As Marshall explained, "We had taken the bacteria and cultured them. We had moved them into the microbiology disease territory. If there was something on a culture plate that you could look at under a microscope, it was real to those people. Straight away you had some allies." Marshall observed that there was a major incentive for the microbiologists to get involved:

> Peptic ulcer was a billion-dollar disease. Tagamet was selling for $2 billion to $3 billion a year. If you couldn't cure cancer, the second best thing would be to treat ulcers. This was a driver for gastroenterology in those days. Everything was funded by ulcer drugs. All of a sudden, people started thinking, "Hey, I'm just a poor penniless microbiologist, but if I could get onto these bacteria and get into the ulcer treatment business with antibiotics, it would fund my whole lab for the next ten years."

Martin Skirrow continued to study the gastric bacteria, as did other scientists in the United States and Australia. Marshall's ideas had the virtue of being easily testable, so some researchers (like Martin Blaser) who originally intended to disprove his hypotheses were brought round by the logic of their own data.

Meanwhile, Marshall, back at home in Perth, was trying to eradicate the microbes in his patients. He discovered that DeNol seemed to work better when it was supplemented with Metronidazole, another antibiotic. After Marshall used both drugs to treat ten patients who had seriously relapsed, eight of them had no further episodes in the six months he was observing them.[24] This was encouraging news, but Marshall said that physicians were still not taken with his ideas. Microbiologists, he explained, had nothing to lose by delving into the study of unusual bacteria. But gastroenterologists thought they already had a good explanation of ulcers—and a treatment. The problem was solved as far as they were concerned. Moreover, Marshall said, "They were in the ulcer business. And although they wouldn't say it, if the ulcers got cured, they'd be out of business. They didn't have an incentive to have a new treatment that actually cured the disease."

Marshall and Warren were still working on what would be their second publication in the *Lancet*. Dr. Warren recalled:

> First of all it was written by Barry. Barry wrote a whole lot of stuff that was very unsatisfactory. It was a huge paper with a whole lot of stuff in it. It wasn't well arranged, but he wanted to get it done as quickly as he could. I just went through and rearranged it all and cut out three-quarters of it. Then I gave it to my wife to read, because she is very good with literature. She could read it. She was a doctor, of course. She could read it through as a professional but she could also read it through, not as a pathologist or gastroenterologist. She could pick up any jargon. We cut out all the jargon. I think Barry's wife did that too.

Marshall agreed with this version of events. He said, laughing, "Our wives wrote that paper." At the end of 1983, they sent off their article about what they were now considering a new bacterium. They tentatively called it "pyloric campylobacter." In 1989, it was renamed *Helicobacter pylori*—"helicobacter" for "a spiral rod" and "pylori" meaning "pertaining to the lower stomach." The *Lancet* had already published their initial letters on the subject, but the first reviewers the journal editor approached with the new piece would not recommend publication. Apparently they did not consider the paper important or interesting enough. A lot was riding on this publication, especially for Marshall. His position as gastroenterology registrar in Fremantle had come to an end. While Ian Hislop had found him a spot in the microbiology department, this too was a short-term placement and he didn't know where he would be working when it ended. He continued to apply for research funding, but had no idea whether it would come through.

Marshall began collaborating with Stewart Goodwin at Royal Perth Hospital on a small study designed to show that the bacteria he had cultured would induce either gastritis or ulcers in an animal. He wanted to demonstrate that the bacteria were *not* secondary to the inflammation, but came first and *caused* the stomach pathology. The plan was to use pigs in the experiment because they develop the same stomach diseases as humans do. To simulate the human situation as much as possible, the pigs were fed food from the hospital kitchen. They were inoculated with the bacteria several times and periodically tested to see if they were infected. A strict schedule was followed. On Thursday evenings they fasted for twelve hours and on Fridays they were scoped. Unfortunately, the pigs turned out to be recalcitrant subjects. It was hard to catch them (they probably figured out the routine pretty quickly) and difficult to anesthetize them. One pig was so stressed by the whole experience that it had a heart attack and had to be resuscitated! Once the pigs reached forty kilograms, they were almost too large for the endoscope to reach their duodenums. But from Marshall's point of view, the worst aspect of the experiment was that no infection could be detected. He abandoned the research.[25]

At the same time, Marshall's efforts to treat patients with ulcers and gastritis continued to garner success. He was able to get rid of the microbes using bismuth in combination with several other antibiotics—amoxicillin, erythromycin, or metronidazole. This still wasn't enough, however, to cause many of his medical colleagues to give up the psychological model of gastric disease. Marshall summed up their attitude this way: "Those patients are all crazy anyway. They are psychosomatic. You tell them, Dr. Marshall, they will be cured with the antibiotics. You are so charismatic, you tell them that and they just feel better. They are totally cured, you take away the stress. It's just like hypnotism." And he characterized his response, too: "I'm impressed that you think I'm so good, but it seems to me it's probably the amoxicillin I'm giving them."

Despite these results, Marshall was growing increasingly frustrated. The animal model hadn't worked out at all. He hadn't proved that the bacteria *caused* ulcers or gastritis. The status quo was holding fast. Marshall's current job would only last until the end of 1984. He had no idea whether a double-blind trial he was planning for 1985 would ever get funded. Furthermore, he was distressed by the fact that some people were still dying of bleeding ulcers and others were being crippled by stomach operations. He remembered one case vividly—a young man who "would just sit there bleeding and bleeding and bleeding. And the surgeons were like, 'Wow, if he doesn't stop bleeding we'll be able to do a total gastrectomy [complete removal of the stomach]. We haven't done one of those in years.' I can remember that case like it was yesterday." Marshall searched for bacteria in the patient's stomach biopsies and couldn't find any. Then he tested the man for antibodies, and he recalled, "That person had antibodies so high I knew that *Helicobacter* were there somewhere. Even if we couldn't see them in the microscope, we needed to get some antibiotics. Not everybody had a harmless *Helicobacter*. Some people reacted very badly to it." Though Marshall had admitted the young man into the hospital, he did not remain in Marshall's care. When Marshall showed his test results to the doctors who were looking after him, they did not prescribe antibiotics, even though Marshall thought it was such a simple thing to try. The patient had a total gastrectomy—something which may have been completely unnecessary. "I was too upset to go back to see him and to this day have never followed up his case further," Marshall wrote.[26]

In May, the *Lancet* finally accepted the paper about gastric bacteria. This was an important milestone for Marshall, a thirty-one-year-old man working in a small hospital in remote Western Australia, far from the medical mainstream. He had no university affiliation or backing from prestigious granting agencies; the recognition was quite a feat. The paper established a strong correlation between the presence of bacteria and gastric disease.[27] It still did not, however, show that the microbes *caused* the disease. Marshall decided that since his animal experiment had foundered, there was only one thing to do—take the bacteria himself and document what happened.

There is, in fact, a rich tradition of doctors willing to experiment on themselves to make a point. In 1900, three US Army physicians, James Carroll, Aristides Agramonte, and Jesse Lazear, allowed themselves to be bitten by mosquitoes during a yellow fever outbreak in the Spanish American War. They wanted to prove that insects transmitted the virus. The experiment was successful, although Lazear died two weeks after he allowed himself to be infected and Carroll suffered long-term complications which led to his death at the age of fifty-three. In 1950, a trio of Australian scientists, Frank Fenner, Frank Macfarlane Burnet, and Ian Clunies Ross, injected themselves with Myxoma virus to prove that it wasn't dangerous for humans. It was then successfully released into the wild to curb Australia's exploding rabbit population.

Even though what Marshall proposed was not without precedent, it still carried some risk—both professional and personal. "The health risk I thought I could manage," said Marshall. He had done a study of a group of healthy men at the Red Cross Blood Donor Clinic in Fremantle. Forty-three percent of them had positive antibodies against *H. pylori*. This indicated they had had an infection at some point, even though most were unaware of this. It looked as though only a minority of people with the gastric bacteria actually got an ulcer; usually, they had no significant symptoms. Marshall thought he could take his chances. An ulcer was a possibility, but it wasn't a certain outcome by any means. In the worst case, he could probably cure himself like he did his patients. "The professional risk I could not control as well, so I did the experiment in semi-secret," Marshall explained. He was worried that his peers might think he was completely crazy and so not trust anything he said. So he didn't advertise what he was going to do—only a few people knew about it. The head of gastroenterology at the hospital, Ian Hislop, had some idea of what was going on. In early June, Marshall showed up at the endoscopy clinic and asked Hislop to perform an endoscopy on him. Before proceeding, he had to establish that he wasn't already infected. "He [Hislop] didn't want to be part of it, really. He did the endoscopy on me. He said, 'Barry, I don't know why I'm doing this on you. And I don't want to know. I don't know what crazy thing you've got planned.' That was the situation. My other boss was the head of microbiology, David McGecky. He kind of knew about it, because he was doing the cultures. He was on board with me pretty much at that point." Marshall did not submit an application to the hospital ethics committee. "If I had submitted an application to the ethics committee to do the experiment, and they had said, 'No,' well I would still have had to do the experiment. And then I would have been in trouble. In retrospect there's a good chance they would have accepted it, but I couldn't be sure."

To infect himself, Marshall used bacteria he obtained from a middle-aged man with mild active gastritis. He had successfully treated him with bismuth and metronidazole, so he was reasonably sure that if the infection did take hold, he would be able to eradicate it the same way. On the morning of June 12, 1984, Marshall stood in his laboratory, wearing his white lab coat, said, "Cheers," then downed 30 ml. of clear liquid containing 100 million *Helicobacter pylori*. It took a bit of willpower to get it down. "It was like swallowing a strange food—a raw egg or a goldfish," he said. A week later, Marshall woke early and vomited. This continued for three or four days, but he was still able to go to work. When he asked Hislop to perform another endoscopy, the biopsy showed he had active inflammation as well as a moderate number of spiral bacteria in his stomach.

This was good news indeed, he thought to himself. But when he told his wife, Adrienne, whom he had so far kept in the dark, she was less enthusiastic. She insisted that Marshall immediately start taking antibiotics—or face eviction from the household! Thus, two weeks after downing his unusual cocktail, Marshall submitted himself once more to an endoscopy. The biopsy showed that by this time, the spiral bacteria were gone. He took the antibiotics anyway to be on the safe side—and save himself from sleeping under a bridge.[28]

One of the notable things about *H. pylori* was that so many people had them without apparently being aware of it. Marshall's experiment gave him insight into why that was. The symptoms of even an acute infection were not so debilitating that people would pay much attention. They weren't aware of having caught a disease with potentially serious effects, and because the chronic infection was common, any manifestations of it were not remarkable. Marshall explained, "People who are having symptoms don't know what it's like to be normal. They are walking around and they have this concept that there are all sorts of foods and things which look okay, but in fact upset your stomach. This person can't drink red wine, this person doesn't like tomatoes, this person can't eat onions. There is this whole folklore about food, there are good ones and bad ones and everyone is different. They say, 'Well you have to be careful what you eat, some things don't agree with you.'" They didn't realize that they could eat whatever they wanted if the infection they had was eradicated. Another factor which helped *H. pylori* escape notice was that it was particularly prevalent among medical professionals. Marshall said, "Doctors and nurses are all infected with *Helicobacter* because nobody realized that secretions in vomit, for example, were infectious. Acid is sterile, you see. Imagine if you were an emergency room nurse for ten years. You'd be touching vomit so many times, you'd be splashing around the place. Anybody in the medical profession ended up infected with *Helicobacter.* A patient would go into a gastroenterologist and tell him about his symptoms, 'Sometimes I have a little meal, but I feel uncomfortable and full.' The doctor, on the other side of the desk would say, 'That's normal, I get that.'"

But as news of Marshall's experiment began to leak out, *H. pylori* was slowly being flushed out of hiding. An American reporter from a tabloid called the *Star* phoned Robin Warren wanting to know more about his research. Marshall said, "I can't remember how they had got on to it. They had some connection to Proctor & Gamble. Proctor & Gamble was starting to leak snippets of information to the general public, saying Pepto-Bismol might be good for ulcers. But the FDA had not signed off on it. So they couldn't do it in an advertising campaign. They started to leak information out to pump their sales. The tabloid heard about it from them." It was five in the morning when the journalist called, and Warren was grumpy at being roused so early. When the reporter asked him how he knew the bacteria weren't harmless, he overstated the case some, blurting out, "I know because Barry Marshall has just infected himself and damn near died." Warren didn't realize that the *Star* was a scurrilous supermarket rag with a dubious reputation. Nevertheless, when the story came out topped by the attention-grabbing headline, "'Guinea-pig' Doctor Discovers New Cure for Ulcers . . . and the Cause," it depicted the research fairly accurately. As a result, thousands of people who did not read the mainstream media heard that there might be help for their stomach problems.

At the end of July, Larry Altman, a doctor and a full-time journalist for the *New York Times*, also wrote about the research. It was reprinted in papers around the world.[29] More people heard the news. Warren recalled:

> Lots of patients wanted to be treated. They had awful pains and most of the treatment was eating milk and chalk and so on—terrible. And the surgical treatment, they might take your stomach out. Things weren't too good for people with chronic ulcer disease. People wanted to be treated. They went to their GPs and demanded to be treated. We used to get letters from GPs asking us how you treat it. We'd tell them. Certainly there was quite a nucleus of GPs, particularly in Perth here, who, I don't know if it was because they were in

> Perth and nearby, but they were particularly interested and were treating the infections. They were quite keen on it. The fact that the specialists weren't interested didn't seem to matter much.

In 1985, Barry Marshall's paper about his self-experimentation appeared in the *Australian Medical Journal*. Marshall did not try to conceal the fact that he was the volunteer who "received pyloric campylobacter by mouth." But, he said, "it wasn't front and centre. It was a little bit of shyness about the experiment, so it was written in the third person." In the paper he recounted, "The subject was one of the writers (B.J.M.), a 32-year old man, a light smoker and social drinker, who had no known gastrointestinal disease or family history of peptic ulceration."[30] Marshall conceived of the experiment because it fulfilled one of Koch's postulates. He had isolated the pathogen from an individual who was sick, grown it, injected it into someone who was healthy, and documented the progress of the disease. Lacking an animal, he had made himself the subject of the experiment. But I wondered whether you could establish causation in another way—by showing that antibiotics were effective against the disease. Koch didn't have antibiotics, but Marshall did. He could demonstrate that if you eliminated the bacteria, patients' symptoms disappeared. When I asked Marshall about this option, he said, "I was also doing that. I had a study starting up, but a double-blind study of one hundred patients takes you three years. You recruit them for a year, follow them up for a year, or longer. At that point, I was impatient, I couldn't wait that long. I thought it was important to get this thing moving. It was a very common disease and people were dying from ulcers all the time. Twenty or thirty people a year in my hospital would die of a peptic ulcer." The story of the young doctor who was so frustrated by the intransigence of the backward medical profession that he made himself ill to make his case had instant appeal. Ulcer patients paid attention. Doctors, too, were struck by this graphic demonstration. Papadimitriou recalled that when he heard about it, he asked himself, "Why didn't I do it?" Then he said:

> I'm being a bit facetious. But I began to think, "Maybe those things were important. Maybe we should have followed things up a bit more." When Barry Marshall started drinking bacterial culture, that to me was, "Hold on a second. These things actually cause a disease. They *are* disease-causing bacteria." Then I could see the links. We

> are still not quite certain as to how the presence of bacteria results in stomach ulceration. It's not by direct invasion. It's because of the cytokines that are secreted and the fact that histamine-like substances get secreted by the bacteria, and they in turn influence the physiological status of hydrochloric-acid-producing cells and so on and so forth. It's not exactly clear how they induce the peptic ulceration. Nevertheless, get rid of them and patients feel better. No doubt about that. It was a major step forward.

Researchers all over the world wanted to see if they could duplicate the Australian results. Warren said, "There was a lot of work published about our work in the two years after we published our original papers. A large percentage of these papers were just repeating the work that we had done. Obviously they were trying to prove that we were wrong. They repeated our work and published it again. It wasn't that they were publishing anything new. They were publishing what we had done in 1984—over and over and over again. Everybody had to do it for themselves."

Arthur Morris, a registrar in pathology at the Auckland Hospital in Auckland, New Zealand, even decided to follow Marshall's example and swallow *H. pylori*. He said during a phone interview from his office in Auckland, "There were elements of Barry's ingestion study that were incomplete." Morris wanted to see whether the bacteria would establish a *chronic* infection and whether antibodies would develop over time. (Marshall hadn't found any, but that may have been because he wasn't infected for very long.) Morris also wanted to measure the acidity of the stomach before and after the microbes had taken hold. Marshall had commented about the fact that his vomit didn't taste acidic. He had also noted that William Osler already described the phenomenon in his book *Principles and Practice of Medicine*, when he wrote about what was, in 1919, apparently a well-known syndrome, "gastritis with hypochlorhydria"—low stomach acid.[31] (The syndrome was subsequently neglected and not included in later textbooks.) However, Marshall hadn't taken any precise measurements of the acid levels in his stomach.

Thus it was that one day in December 1985 Morris was lying on a table in the Auckland Hospital waiting for Gordon Nicholson, a gastroenterologist, to scope his stomach to make sure that he had no infection. Morris recalled:

> Nicholson had gone and spoken to another doctor, an expert on infectious diseases. He had said, "I think to be on the safe side, you guys should go to the ethical committee and get it signed off." So we went to the ethical committee and they virtually washed their hands of it. They didn't say, "No." That was helpful. They said if I'm doing it with my eyes open and without duress it was over to us. Then they said they thought the proposed study had no scientific value, no scientific merit. I strongly disagreed with that. There is a long history of ingesting gastrointestinal pathogens under controlled circumstances in medical microbiology and infectious diseases. So there is a strong precedent for it. If they genuinely felt there was no merit, they should have said, "No," but they didn't. They said, "You're a big boy; if you've got your eyes open, and no one is forcing you to do it, then it's over to you to do it. I got an ethical sign off—sort of—and then we proceeded.

First, Morris drank a culture which he obtained from Marshall's lab in Perth. As Barry Marshall had done, Morris suspended the bacteria in alkaline peptone water (a medium used for growing bacteria). "Its taste was not pleasant, but I got it down before the taste really was appreciated." No infection resulted, unfortunately, so he tried again six weeks later with bacteria obtained from a patient at his own hospital. He said, "The taste was a put-off and this made the second ingestion more daunting. I gagged a few times after swallowing it. I was a bit concerned that I might bring it back up but that didn't happen."

This time an acute infection took hold. Morris had a lot of abdominal pain and couldn't sleep. In fact, he was so sore, he wondered whether he might have a bowel obstruction. But after a week or so, the symptoms subsided. The bacteria, though, firmly established themselves in his stomach. They were still there at day 67 when he began one month of treatment with bismuth subsalicylate. A biopsy at day 103 showed no bacteria and almost complete resolution of the stomach inflammation. "However," Morris recalled, "about nine months later, all the data were coming in that monotherapy [treatment with one drug] probably didn't work. To see what was happening almost a year after the original ingestion, I repeated the biopsies and *H. pylori* was everywhere." Morris treated himself four times with single-agent antibiotics unsuccessfully. Then on day 966, he used a combination of antibiotics and bismuth that rid him of the microbes. An endoscopy 106 days later revealed that the mixture had worked. There was no *H. pylori* to be seen, and the gastritis was gone.[32]

Morris had shown what Marshall had not—that the bacteria could cause a stubborn *chronic* infection. He'd done what he set out to do. He observed, "Even if Barry had shown everything, reproducibility is an important bit of science. It would have been a bit more of a me-too study, but it would have cemented the original observation." Would he have any hesitation about doing something like that again? He said, "I think later on, when the association with gastric carcinoma became more obvious and the difficulties with eradicative therapy were fully understood, volunteer studies became more questionable. I would have a lot more reservations about it. It was done in a window of ignorance."

Despite the flood of research confirming Marshall's and Warren's original results, medical practice changed slowly. Marshall explained:

> In my Nobel lecture I had this quote from Dan Boorstin [an American historian, lawyer, and, for twelve years, the head of the Library of Congress]. He had this saying that the reason people don't accept new things is not from ignorance; it's the illusion of knowledge. Everybody knew that stress caused ulcers, they didn't need another explanation. The whole community, all the patients, all the doctors, they all knew that stress caused ulcers. They didn't need to have bacteria—that was just a complicating issue. And it was extra work, once you started worrying about *Helicobacter*. If you have to see thirty patients a day to keep your salary up, when the ulcer patient comes in, you just write, "Cimetidine or Tagamet, five repeats." Here you go, out the door. That's ulcer. Whereas the new one: "It could be this bacteria, let's get a blood test. If it's positive, we have to give you those antibiotics. Then we'll give you a breath test." You can see there are all kinds of activities that now go on to cure a patient. The patient is very interested in this new technology, but the doctor is not.

The breath test that Marshall mentions was developed in 1985. It relies on *H. pylori*'s ability to create a non-acidic microclimate around itself. The bacterium converts urea, which is abundant in the stomach, into ammonia and carbon dioxide. This produces a change in a person's breath which can be easily detected by a simple test that a doctor can run in his office. While doctors may have initially been reluctant to order up yet another test for their patients, it actually did help push

Marshall's ideas forward. More accurate than blood tests, and both cheaper and less invasive than an endoscopy, the breath test was a remarkably convenient way of diagnosing the presence of *H. pylori*. Because physicians had such a useful tool and were able to offer effective antibiotic treatments, their opinions gradually started to shift. When the conventional anti-acids were not working, or when their patients relapsed, some doctors would try the new cures. Marshall said, "The only thing that made any difference to them was when they treated their own patients in a clinical trial of one and got a good result. They would switch over."

THE INTERESTING RELATIONSHIP BETWEEN *H. PYLORI* INFECTION AND GASTRIC CANCERS

In March 1986, Marshall took a position as professor of medicine at the University of Virginia and moved to the United States with his family. He was, he writes, "expecting to find a receptive audience in the United States."[33] But his ideas were not officially sanctioned for another eight years. In February 1994, the National Institutes of Health in the US issued a "consensus statement" declaring that *H. pylori* was a gastrointestinal pathogen and that ulcer patients infected with the microbes needed antibiotics as well as anti-acids. The statement also said, "The interesting relationship between *H. pylori* infection and gastric cancers requires further exploration."[34]

The notion that there might be such an interesting relationship was not original. In 1918, James Ewing, a famous American pathologist, wrote a review on the subject. He found suggestions that stomach cancer and ulcers might be linked going back as far as 1840. After looking at the evidence, he concluded that "the cancerous transformation of peptic ulcer is rather infrequent."[35] Marshall had referred to this possibility in his original letter to the *Lancet*, and Warren had noticed experimental evidence supporting it. Warren told me, "An interesting thing I'd seen was that patients with cancer in the stomach seemed to have the same changes in the surrounding mucosa, around the cancer, as patients with very severe, long-standing inflammation. I began wondering if the infection could be causing the cancer. I had no other evidence for it. I had no statistical evidence. It looked reasonable and it looked logical." Marshall and Warren did not find the statistical evidence that was needed. They left it up to others. One of those was David Forman.

David Forman is now the head of the Cancer Information Section at the International Agency for Research on Cancer in Lyons, France. When I interviewed him by phone at his office there, he told me that in the mid-eighties he was working at Oxford University in the field of cancer epidemiology. "I'd been asked by my then-boss to work on stomach cancer. We were following it up in terms of gastritis, the inflammation, and asking the question, 'Well, if inflammation causes stomach cancer, what causes inflammation in the first place?' We were largely following dietary hypotheses." It so happened that Richard Smallwood, a visiting professor of gastroenterology from Australia, had an office in the same building as Forman. The two men met, and Smallwood told Forman about two Australian investigators who had isolated a bacterium that appeared to live in the stomach and to cause gastritis. He said that in his opinion it was exciting work, well worth looking at. But when Forman first heard about it, it seemed like a "totally crazy hypothesis." Forman explained that to understand his position, you had to "wind the clock back thirty years." At that time, only a few scientists were looking for infectious causes of cancer and those who did were focused on viruses or parasites responsible for rare cancers in developing countries. Many researchers had been thinking about how chemical and dietary exposures might explain stomach cancer. The idea that they could be wrong about such a common malignancy—that bacteria might be a major causal influence—seemed "very radical," according to Forman. He went on:

> The stomach was regarded, because of the acidity there, as an organ which didn't harbor bacteria. The environment would be too hostile to keep the bacterial colonization alive. Consequently, bacteria were thought to exist in the lower gut but not in the upper gut. At that point, the whole concept just went against conventional thinking—not that anyone had really nailed down the major causes of gastric cancer. The idea that it could be bacteria, which were not thought to reside in the stomach, made it seem even more left field.

Furthermore, the Australian ideas seemed to fly in the face of what was known about the epidemiology of stomach cancer. Forman said, "Duodenal ulcers were largely associated with relative affluence and the pressures of living in modern society. There was this whole story that they were largely stress-induced, whereas stomach cancer was seen as a disease of social deprivation and poverty." In other words, ulcers then were seen as a disease of the rich, and stomach cancer a disease of the poor. Against this epidemiological background, the suggestion that the two conditions were associated and might have a common cause didn't make sense.

Forman decided to disprove these new ideas about cancer and stomach bacteria. He used blood samples from a couple of large studies originally done during an investigation of cardiovascular disease. Since these studies recorded what caused the participants' deaths, Forman could go back and test samples from the individuals who developed gastric cancer. Then he could see whether they had higher levels of *Helicobacter* antibodies (prior to developing the cancer) than the control group, which remained disease-free. He concluded that between 35 percent and 55 percent of all gastric cancers might be associated with *H. pylori* infection.[36] That same year a couple of American studies with similar results were also published. Martin Blaser, the erstwhile *H. pylori* skeptic, published a paper which looked at a cohort of about six thousand Japanese Americans living in Hawaii. It determined that *H. pylori* was "strongly associated with an increased risk of stomach cancer."[37] Julie Parsonnet, a researcher at Stanford, looked at a group of Californians and found that *H. pylori* might be a co-factor in the development of some gastric cancers.[38] Forman said, "We all latched on to this lead at the same time." Forman became a convert to Marshall's way of thinking. He said, "I guess it was the effect of having positive results ourselves and having them confirmed rapidly by other groups with independent methods. Those studies in combination were very influential—they were pivotal."

In 1994, Forman took part in the World Health Organization (WHO) deliberations about *H. pylori*. Twenty experts from around the world met in Lyons at the International Agency for Cancer Research and had what Forman described as an "intense debate." In the end, they declared that *H. pylori* was definitely a carcinogen for humans. But even at this stage of the game, Forman said, "There was quite a lot of dissent. The Japanese reps at that meeting dissented from the decision and wanted their dissent minuted." The monograph detailing the conclusion of the meeting noted that Dr. Tomoyuki Shirai, a pathologist from Nagoya City University Medical School in Japan, "disassociated himself from the overall evaluation."[39] Forman explained, "At the time, Japan had some of the highest stomach cancer rates in the world. There was a lot of Japanese research going on into stomach cancer, but because none of this *Helicobacter* research had been undertaken in Japan, our Japanese colleagues were much less willing than others to accept this change in mindset." Nevertheless, the WHO's evaluation of *H. pylori* soon became the approved position. It was official—a bacterium was a cause of stomach cancer.

Just over ten years later, at five p.m. on the evening of October 4, Robin Warren and Barry Marshall were having dinner together in Perth. Warren said, "My phone went. When I answered it, a man said, 'This is Stockholm calling.' 'Yes,' I thought, 'Tell me another one.' When he finally convinced me who he was and that I'd won the Nobel Prize, he said, 'You can't say anything because the official announcement is not for half an hour. You can't tell anybody.' I asked him, 'Can I tell Barry? He's sitting opposite me.' The man from Stockholm said, 'No, no, you can't tell him.' I asked, 'Can I give him the phone, and you tell him?' I didn't know what the difference was, but that's what I did, I handed him the phone. He told Barry."

The two Australian scientists had come to the end of the long road to the Nobel.

5

PAUL EWALD STALKS THE STEALTH INFECTIONS

Darwin's probably my biggest hero.

—Paul Ewald

THIS THING COULD BE MANIPULATING ME

My next stop was in Kentucky—Louisville, "Loo uh vul," if you're speaking as the locals do. It was September 2011, and still languorously hot. As I walked from the bed and breakfast where I was staying to the University of Louisville campus, I found myself seeking shade. I had come to meet Paul Ewald; we were going to have a couple of interviews. He was not a medical doctor; nevertheless, his work forms an important part of the new way of thinking about cancer and infections. It helps us to see not just that pathogens are linked to malignancies, but *why* this is so.

I met Ewald at his office—cement block construction, no pictures on the walls, desks piled high with books and papers. Though the room was utilitarian, it was bright; a window looked out over lush trees and the busy campus. Ewald is an evolutionary biologist and a key figure in what is called Darwinian medicine—the application of modern evolutionary theory to our understanding of health and disease. Traditionally, a medical investigator would look at the problem of cancer and try to explain why one person got sick and another didn't. An evolutionary

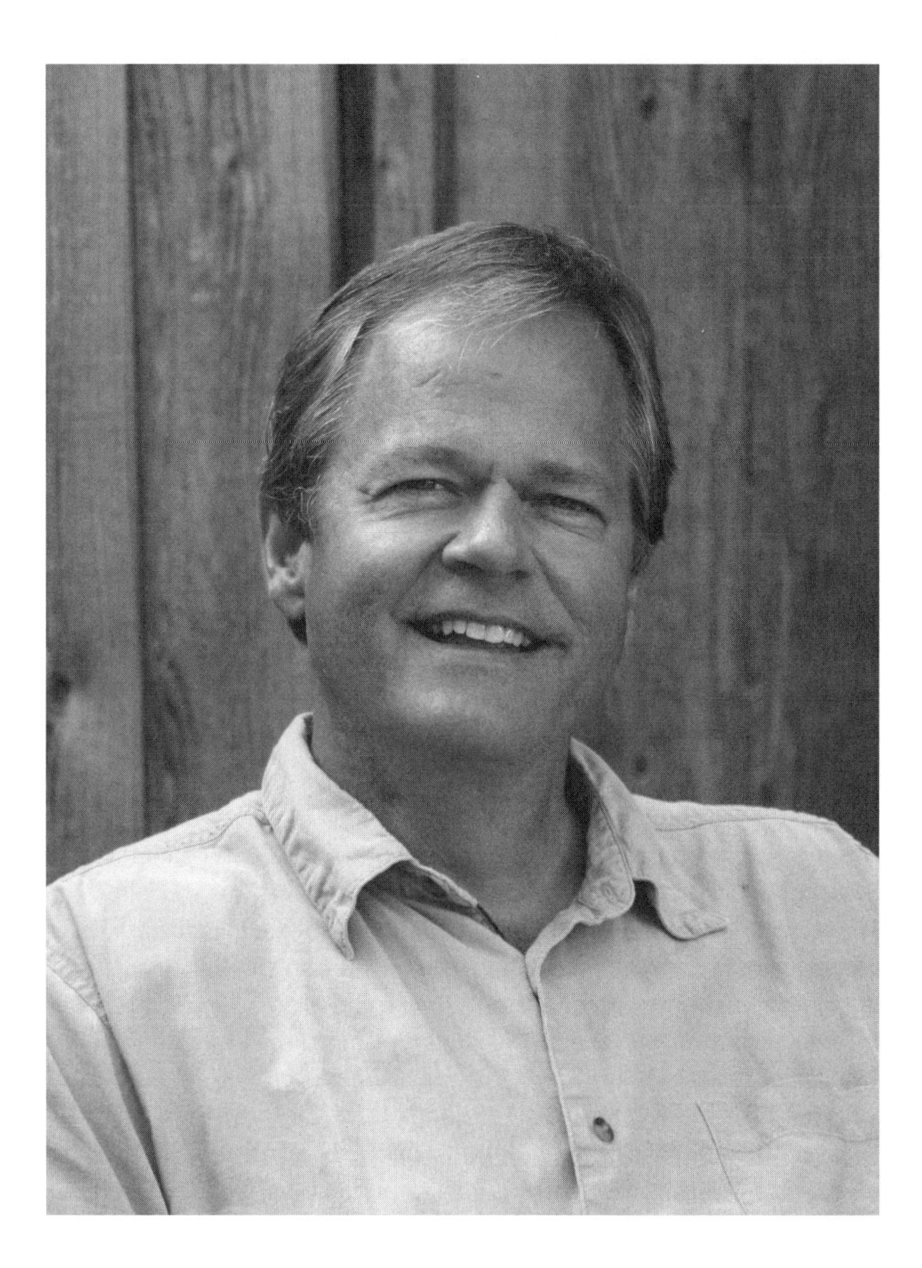

Figure 5.1. Paul Ewald. Photo courtesy of Holly A. Swain Ewald

biologist would ask how natural selection can help us understand why human beings *in general* are vulnerable to cancer.

Sometimes called a visionary, Ewald is famous for asking provocative questions. In 2008, he gave a TED Talk called "Can We Domesticate Germs?" He argued that we should not be thinking about eradicating pathogens, but about making them less dangerous. He believes conventional ideas about chronic diseases are wrong-headed. While many people consider that these illnesses are caused by genetic predispositions, bad lifestyle choices, or chemical stresses, Ewald is convinced infections are often wholly or partially to blame. If he's right, sweeping changes to medicine, the way we treat and prevent many sicknesses, are in order. This is a man about whom there is considerable intellectual buzz, but in person, he is friendly and helpful. His instructions to me about how to find his office were minutely detailed. *Scientific American* and the *Atlantic Monthly* have both published articles about him. Ewald is himself the author of two books, *The Evolution of Infectious Diseases* and *Plague Time: How Stealth Infections Cause Cancers, Heart Disease, and Other Deadly Ailments*. With his wife, Holly Swain Ewald, he recently wrote a third book, *Controlling Cancer*. As you will see, his road to that subject was long and winding, and it grew out of a deep understanding of our relationship to pathogens.

Ewald and I talked for several hours about his research and his family. He told me that he began writing papers together with Holly, who has a PhD in neuroscience, about four years ago. They met in 2002 when Ewald was invited to give a talk on March 20 at Bard College in New York, where Holly was working in a biology lab. A terrible late-season blizzard hit just as Ewald set out; he said, "Any sensible person wouldn't have gone to give this seminar." Ewald went anyway, creeping along the highway at thirty miles an hour. He was four hours late, but managed to be in time to take in a presidential dinner and give his talk—about schizophrenia and infection. Holly came up to him afterward, and said, "I thought this would be an old story about cytomegalovirus, and that it was going to be far-fetched, but I think you're on the right track." They ended up talking and never stopped. Ewald said, "It was the first day of spring or the last day of winter, I can't remember which. Both of us were in sort of a winter period of our lives and so I came out of the blizzard and it was the end of winter and the beginning of spring. It's a nice story. We knew that we wanted to get married within a month or so. I had been married before and we had separated two years earlier."

Ewald is tall, tanned, and fit; he rides his bicycle to the campus every day—a distance of about four miles. He and his wife recently bought a property in the country where they keep three horses. Their current project is to fence the entire forty acres using fallen cedars. To cut them down to size, they use an old-fashioned crosscut saw. It's much quieter than a chain saw, said Ewald, and allows him to observe animals and birds. He told me that not long ago, he and Holly were out sawing when he happened to look up and see a large deer standing quietly behind her, quite unperturbed. "I think we were on its path, and it wondered what we were doing there," he said. Ewald told me that birds were his first scientific love, and he still finds them intriguing although he hasn't been doing any research in that field since the mid-1990s. For now pathogens are all-consuming.

As an undergraduate at the University of California at Irvine and later as a graduate student at the University of Washington, Ewald was particularly interested in the aggressive behavior of birds. Why were some more belligerent than others? He investigated hummingbirds, gulls, sparrows, red-winged blackbirds. In an early paper, he explained that while dominant birds could get the food they wanted easily, they paid a price—expending more energy fighting. Subordinates, on the other hand, didn't clash so much; both strategies had costs and benefits. It wasn't clear that the domineering birds won out in evolutionary terms—that they had more offspring than those at the bottom of the pecking order.[1] In other words, nature was supporting two approaches. As we will see later, Ewald made use of that principle again in another context.

Ewald was making valuable discoveries about bird behavior, and he might have happily continued in this vein, but for something that aroused his curiosity while he was on an excursion to Kansas. It was January 1977, and he had come to study Harris's sparrow. While he was on the field trip, the focus of his scientific inquiry expanded. Like Sir Isaac Newton, who saw an apple fall to the ground and started on a train of thought which led him to formulate the Law of Universal Gravitation, Ewald had a perfectly mundane experience which led him to far-reaching and unexpected conclusions.

For Ewald, it was a bad case of diarrhea. At first, he thought, "I'll let my body take care of it." It was, after all, the seventies, and natural remedies were in vogue. But then he had another thought: "This thing could be manipulating me. It could be that I'm trying to get rid of the organism, but it could also be that the organism is manipulating me for its own dispersal." As he explained, "If the manifestation were a defense, you wouldn't want to treat it. But if it were a manipulation by the pathogen, then treating the diarrhea would help to control the organism's spread." Which was it? When he got back to Irvine, he went to the library to find out—to satisfy his personal curiosity. It was the start of a long quest to understand the evolution of pathogens and what that means for us.

IT TIES EVERYTHING TOGETHER

Paul Ewald was born in September 1953 and grew up in Wilmette, a lakeside community about fifteen miles north of Chicago. His father, Arno Ewald, was a physics professor at Northwestern University, and his mother, Sara, taught psychology at a nearby teachers' college. Ewald has written about his mother, about her strong resistance to infections and the fact that she has aged more slowly than other people. He clearly admires her. He said, "My mother is very smart and incredibly considerate and thoughtful in her interactions with people. Until you get to know her, you don't realize how smart she is because she is so nice to people." When she was seventy-nine, he recalled, she was hit by a truck. It crushed her pelvis and collapsed her lungs. The doctors didn't think she was going to make it. But she was very determined. Arno had died a few years before, and she had just met another man who interested her. She really wanted to get better. A month after her accident she was getting out of bed, two months later she was walking with a cane, and three months later she was off to Europe with the new love of her life.

Ewald has two children in their twenties, and I asked him if they shared his interests. He said that his son was studying political science but his daughter, Sarah, "ended up in biology, amazingly enough." He recalled,

> I always worried tremendously about her. In high school, everything out of her mouth was a criticism. She was too cool for studies. One time I was trying to help her on math. She said, "I can't do it, I can't do it." I said, "Just look at this. I know you can do it." She said, "I can't! I can't!" I told her, "If you take that attitude, you'll spend your

> life flipping burgers at McDonald's." She just got so mad, stomped off muttering, "Flipping burgers in McDonalds!" She was so angry, so livid. I think that stuck with her, though I could be making too much out of it. She got really focused on studying in her last year of undergraduate. She applied to graduate school and got in everywhere. Then she went to Berkeley. She did some good work, published a paper in *Nature*, and graduated. Holly and I, and my ex-wife, went. She got the award for the best thesis in molecular biology.

And then Ewald's eyes welled up with tears, and he stopped for a moment to catch his composure. He went on to tell me that Sarah now has a fellowship at Stanford and like him, studies cancer. "She's got more expertise in immunology than I do. I ask her about that."

Ewald was the youngest of four boys. He said, "I was always competing with my older brothers. I was very influenced by my brother who was five years older. He would do things that I would want to try because he was doing them." When Paul's brother Steve was in high school, he began doing push-ups to stay in shape. Paul, who was then in about the fifth grade, did them too; he kept on going until he couldn't do any more. When his brother did sit-ups he followed suit. Paul remembered that once when Steve did about fifty sit-ups, he said to Paul, "See if you can do fifty." Paul got to fifty and then, exercising his own fierce determination, kept on going, and going, and going. "I went to 2,000," he said. "I was always a little bit over the top in these things," he added somewhat ruefully.

As a youngster, Ewald collected insects and learned about their natural history. He memorized the names of the different geological periods. "I was always getting books out and reading them," he said, "I had this sense that I wanted to read all the books in the library." But he didn't work that hard in high school. He got mostly Bs (except in math, where he earned As). Ewald recounted, "I had a girlfriend. I was much more interested in spending time with her. She was not very studious, a year younger than me." After graduation, Ewald went to the University of California at Irvine, about forty miles south of Los Angeles. His academic career did not start auspiciously. He got Ds on his first midterms. "I didn't know how to take those multiple-choice exams. I actually worked hard on how to take tests. I told myself, 'Don't overthink the questions. Figure out what they are trying to ask you and answer in that way.'" Once he got the hang of it, he started to get As. Ewald had not chosen a career, but he enrolled as a biology major. Early in his studies, he was struck by the explanatory power of the theory of evolution. He said, "I remember deciding in the first semester, 'Wow, this is really interesting because it ties everything together.' Darwin's probably my biggest hero. His work was so broadly relevant. It probably explains life on other planets as well." In Ewald's second year, his girlfriend came out west to join him. They lived together for a year and a half on the beach. "That can make a person prone to not doing your school work," he reflected. It didn't suit him and he and his girlfriend began to have conflicts. He told her, "I've got to do well. I can't just sit on the beach drinking wine. I've got to do this work." The relationship deteriorated and they broke up.

In Ewald's final year as an undergraduate, Lynn Carpenter, an ecologist and biologist, was his mentor. When I phoned her at her home in southern California, she told me that under her supervision, Ewald wrote a paper about the territoriality of hummingbirds, showing how their aggression was influenced by the amount of food that was available. It required painstaking dawn-to-dusk observations. Carpenter recalled that when they had to know which bird owned a territory and which one was a poacher, Ewald cleverly figured out how to distinguish them. She said, "From a distance, when a bird would be hovering at the feeder, he would shoot it with a little bit of paint and use different colors in different patterns so he could tell individuals apart. That was very ingenious. It meant that we didn't have to disturb them by trying to net them."

Ewald applied to graduate school at the University of Washington. Its ecology program was one of the most demanding in the country. Generally only four out of about three hundred applicants were accepted. Ewald was on a waiting list when the faculty decided to make an exception and take on one more student. Ewald got in—on the strength of his paper about hummingbirds.

WHY DOES THE PATHOGEN DO THIS?

Ewald began writing a thesis about aggression in hummingbirds. But he had not forgotten his questions about diarrheal diseases. To his surprise, the answers he was seeking weren't readily available in the library; no one else seemed to be thinking about these issues the way he was. So he proceeded on his own to try to figure out what was going on. "I had learned that any biological question is not well understood unless you think in terms of the Why and the How. The Why is the evolutionary question—why does a characteristic allow the organism to survive and reproduce better in competition with others? The How is the mechanistic question—how does it work?" Ewald explained that if you wanted to understand cholera from a mechanistic point of view, you would look at how the bacterium makes a toxin which enters the cells in the intestinal walls of the host. Then you would describe how the toxin changes the cells' physiology and disrupts the normal flow of sodium and chloride. This causes large amounts of fluid to accumulate (up to twenty liters a day in an untreated person!). It has to go somewhere and so you get diarrhea. But the other, more complicated question is, "*Why* does the pathogen do this?" To find the answer you have to consider that the large intestine is teeming with organisms—all competing with cholera for resources. The gush of liquid enables the cholera bacterium to wash away its rivals. It can attach itself to the walls of the host's intestine, but other organisms cannot. So while the cholera hangs on in the torrent, its competition is swept away. Then the cholera can reproduce, unhampered by other contenders, and ride another surge of liquid to disperse in the environment.

As Ewald realized from the start, symptoms are complicated. In the paper he wrote about all of this, "Evolutionary Biology and the Treatment of Signs and Symptoms of Infectious Disease," he explained that they arise out of a tug-of-war between hosts and pathogens. But their *function* isn't always obvious and sometimes may surprise us. Though we tend to regard fever as an unpleasant side effect of being sick, it may sometimes be part of the body's defense system. Drawing on animal studies, Ewald pointed to pathogens that break down in high temperatures. Rabbits infected with *Pastuerella multocida* (which attacks their upper respiratory system) have better survival rates if a fever is allowed to run its course than if the high temperature is reduced. He also suggested that diarrhea might sometimes be a cooperative production that benefits both the pathogen and the host. In that case, the losers are the healthy (but susceptible) people who catch the illness because of the germs the diarrhea spreads around.[2]

Ewald's ideas didn't have the impact on medicine that he was hoping for: "Now people are more hesitant about treating fever but even that isn't quite what I would like to see happening." He wanted researchers to create experiments that would answer some of the questions he had raised—to compare the outcome of treating symptoms with that of leaving them unchecked. "They haven't been done," he said, shaking his head. "I thought we would have all this research and figure it out. Then we'd have policy. But it hasn't happened." Nevertheless, the 1980 paper about signs and symptoms helped Ewald, who had just received his PhD, make his academic name. Bruce Fleury teaches evolutionary biology at Tulane University in New Orleans. When I spoke to him on the phone about Paul Ewald, he said that he broke new ground with his work on sign and symptoms. "If he is standing on the shoulders of giants, I have not encountered them yet. As far as I know, he's it."

THE VECTOR-BORNE DISEASES ARE SIGNIFICANTLY MORE SEVERE

Ewald had become interested in another big question: why are some disease organisms more harmful than others? He wasn't satisfied with the usual answer—that as pathogens adapt to new hosts they become milder. This was the doctrine of "commensalism," popular in medicine since the 1930s. The most famous textbook example occurred in Australia when a dozen pairs of rabbits were released in 1859. They multiplied—well, like rabbits—and a hundred years later, 300 million bunnies were devastating the local flora. The Australian government fought back by introducing the South American *Myxoma virus* to the continent. It proved deadly for the rabbits—at first. Their population plummeted by 99 percent, but after a few years it rebounded. The rabbits developed resistance to the virus; the virus also became milder. Ewald told me that when syphilis moved from the New World to the Old World, it seemed to follow the same pattern, striking its early victims with ferocity and later becoming less destructive. Since microbes didn't actually benefit by killing off their hosts, a relatively peaceful co-existence was supposed to develop. It sounded reasonable, but Ewald was skeptical. He thought, "From an evolutionary point of view, you realize that the idea [of a pathogen necessarily evolving to mildness] does not flow logically out of the idea of natural selection."

In order to reproduce, germs need to move from one organism to another; they need an exit strategy. Ewald thought that a pathogen which normally passes directly from person to person would have few opportunities for infection if its host was immobile, confined to bed. It would do better if its victim was ambulatory. He hypothesized that for such microbes, the cost of virulence was high and milder variants (which allowed their victims to move around their community) would tend to become more common. Commensalism was likely. But it was not so likely if viruses were carried by mosquitoes. In that case, if microbes grievously weakened their hosts and left them in a delirious fever, unable to walk amongst their fellows, the viruses still had an exit path—insects. Moreover, the more extensively the microbes spread through the circulatory system of their victims, the more likely it was that a mosquito biting one of them would pick up a pathogen along with its meal of blood. Truly debilitated patients would be too exhausted to wave away roving mosquitoes. They'd end up with more bites, increasing the possibility of transmission. In these conditions, Ewald hypothesized that natural selection favored virulence.

Ewald said, "It turned out that vector-borne diseases really are significantly more severe." Diseases transmitted by mosquitoes, like malaria, sleeping sickness, and yellow fever, are among our nastiest. Ewald had used the evolutionary lens to show us why and, in the process, exposed a flaw in a widely held assumption. The mode of transmission that a microbe uses explains a lot about disease; it determines which variants—mild or lethal—come to dominate. When Ewald was studying birds, he had seen that being on top of the pecking order had its costs and benefits, as did being on the bottom. Both strategies had their place. Pathogens weren't that different. Ewald published this research in a paper called "Host-Parasite Relations, Vectors, and the Evolution of Disease Severity."[3]

In 1980, Ewald became a fellow at the University of Michigan. At that time two highly respected biologists were also there—George Williams and Bill Hamilton, founding fathers of Darwinian or evolutionary medicine. Though Charles Darwin had written *On the Origin of Species* in 1859, it had taken more than a hundred years for scientists to begin seriously and systematically considering the implications of his ideas for medicine. George Williams was famous for pushing the gene-centric view of evolution later popularized by Richard Dawkins in *The Selfish Gene*, and for making major contributions to our understanding of aging. Bill Hamilton, considered one of the most important biologists of the twentieth century, was noted for his groundbreaking work on the genetic basis for altruism. "It was a wonderful place to be doing this kind of work," recalled Ewald.

In 1983, Ewald took a job at Amherst College in Massachusetts. By then married, with one daughter, he bought a heritage house built in 1760. It was in need of repair, and he did much of the work himself. He found that often his best ideas came to him while doing manual labor on the house, and he learned to keep a small notebook in his pocket for those flashes of insight. Although Ewald had not started his career in biology with the aim of researching the ecology of pathogens, he was immersing himself in the study of their modes of transmission. It turned out to be a topic with great explanatory potential.

Ewald got interested in an issue which he described to me as a "spinoff" from the project about insect vectors. "I had written," he recalled, "that for diarrheal diseases we have an analog to vector-borne transmission. Water will move pathogens from people who can't move. Attendants take soiled bed sheets and wash them. If the water used for laundry contaminates the drinking supply, then even a person who is confined to bed can infect thousands of others." Ewald surmised that if the diarrheal organisms were like the mosquito-borne microbes, then they ought to be more harmful when water-borne, and milder when transmitted from person-to-person. If this were true, he realized, there was an interesting corollary that could also be tested. "If you clean up the water supplies, you should block the transmission that is independent of host health and mobility. If the only way you're allowing transmission is through mobile people, you ought to cause those organisms to be mild." Paul Ewald was contemplating using what we know about evolution to "de-fang" microbes. Was it really possible to do this, and by such relatively simple methods as improving the water supply?

To answer these questions, Ewald went to the London School of Hygiene and Tropical Medicine on a NATO research fellowship in 1984. The school is a venerable institution; its archives are a treasure trove of information about many infectious diseases. Ewald was interested in its hundred-year-old records about the outbreaks of diarrheal diseases which registered both the types of pathogens involved and whether they were waterborne. Ewald had a vivid sense of being at the crossroads of medical history. Dr. John Snow, who proved that cholera was spread by contaminated water and is considered by many to be the father of modern epidemiology, had opened an office on Frith Street in 1838. This was just a ten-minute walk from the archives where Ewald was doing his research. The same year that Dr. Snow moved to Frith Street, Ewald's great hero, Charles Darwin, had also rented a house on nearby Gower Street. Ewald said:

> They had overlapped just for a year or so. Maybe they had even walked past each other, who knows? The father of epidemiology and the father of evolutionary biology, formulating their ideas right at the same time. It was all in the 1840s. Then I realized I'm linking these two people. I'm doing evolutionary epidemiology. I'm sitting here in this library 130 years later, finally making the connection that John and Charles would have made if they had just sat down and talked—these two brilliant people, two of the great figures in history.

One day Ewald was on the London Tube daydreaming a little about the two men he admired so much and thinking what a privilege it was to be where he was. He looked up and saw the Vauxhall stop. The tracks were elevated at that point, and Ewald gazed out through the window. He realized he was seeing the very same neighborhood where John Snow had done his seminal research. "You look back over your life and ask, 'What were the coolest times?' That, to me, was one of the highlights. It was just about the coolest. I started laughing. People probably thought I was crazy." As Ewald told me how evolutionary epidemiology had captivated him, I was reminded that while logic and rationality are obviously part of science, passion is too.

The research Ewald did in London helped to convince him he was on the right track. He writes: "As water supplies were purified in cholera-endemic regions in India during the 1950s and 1960s, the milder agent of cholera, the El Tor type of *Vibrio cholerae*, displaced the more dangerous form, classical *V. cholerae*. In Bangladesh, however, where the war of independence and extensive socioeconomic difficulties have delayed water purification, classical *V. cholerae* persists."[4] Later another "natural experiment" gave him more evidence. In January 1991, a cholera epidemic arrived in Peru and spread throughout Central and

South America within a couple of years. Ewald told me, "So in Chile within ten years, well really within five years, the bacterium was dominated by strains that were not producing as much toxin as earlier." By contrast, in countries with more polluted water, like Ecuador, the organisms became more detrimental.

Ewald's idea that we can domesticate germs by changing their method of transmission aroused a vigorous debate. That we can domesticate germs is not really at issue. We already do this when we make what are called attenuated or weakened vaccines. They are usually produced by culturing generations of microbes in an artificial environment which is different from the human body. For instance, you might grow a virus at a cool temperature. The viruses that do well are selected and allowed to reproduce. These strains are not likely to flourish—to reproduce quickly—in warm conditions. When introduced into a human, the immune system is able to kill them all easily. However, in most respects, the tamed viruses are similar to the "wild" ones. So the antibodies a human body produces to dispatch them are equally effective against their untamed cousins.

Still scientists wonder whether we can reliably tame germs *outside* a laboratory. Can we make them mild enough to improve health? To prove that it's possible, Ewald would like to do an experiment. "We could introduce clean water supplies for two villages, but not for another two villages. We'll see whether we get the milder strains. It's a great experiment. It's ethically okay because if you have $5 million you could do two villages, but you can't do four. So what you're doing is keeping track of the two where you actually put in the clean water and the two where you don't." Ewald believes forcing the pathogens to depend on mobile hosts for transmission should encourage them to evolve toward mildness. It's virtually a no-risk experiment. Even if the microbes don't become less harmful, at the very least you improve the water supply—a good thing in itself.

INFECTION WAS PLAYING A BIGGER ROLE THAN I HAD THOUGHT

As Ewald put a kettle on for tea, a brass band played loudly on the road below in preparation for a State of the University Address, and professors in colorful academic gowns were crossing the campus, converging for the speech. Ewald started telling me about a maverick thinker called Gregory Cochran. A physicist by training, Cochran became interested in genetics and biology and today is an adjunct professor of anthropology at the University of Utah. "Gregory influenced me quite a bit," Ewald said. "I've always been interested in this issue of infection and cancer, but I think he forced me to think harder about it. I came to the conclusion that infection was playing a bigger role than I had thought previously."

Ewald collaborated with Cochran on a few papers and then in 2000 published his book, *Plague Time: How Stealth Infections Cause Cancers, Heart Disease, and Other Deadly Ailments*. His central idea was that if you think about the evolutionary forces shaping pathogens, you will understand why they play a role in many more diseases than we usually blame them for. He started the book with the observation that causes of disease fall into three categories: "One is bad genes. Another comprises harmful non-infectious aspects of the environment such as radiation, noxious chemicals, and dietary imbalances. The third is infectious damage caused by viruses, bacteria, and other parasites."[5]

Scrutiny of environmental factors has the longest history. In 400 BC, the Greek physician, Hippocrates, suggested in *On Airs, Water, and Places* that "whoever wishes to investigate medicine properly" should look to "the winds," the "quality of the waters," and the "mode" in which people live—"their pursuits, whether they are fond of drinking and eating to excess, and given to indolence, or are fond of exercise and labor, and not given to excess in eating and drinking."[6]

The germ theory of disease came into its own when Robert Koch and Louis Pasteur each articulated it in the late 1800s. Following their work, other scientists found many more disease-causing microbes. They began with illnesses that had obvious symptoms (coughs, sneezes, skin rashes) and "conspicuous transmission chains" (a person became sick soon after direct contact with someone who was already ill).[7] Even a layperson could see what was going on. That's why measles was known to be infectious a century before Dr. Thomas Peebles isolated the virus in 1954, during an outbreak in a private school in Boston. Infections were harder to spot if the pathogens were carried by vectors—water or insects. Significantly trickier were situations where considerable time elapsed between the initial exposure and the appearance of problems.

Nevertheless, with new tools and methods, investigators began tracking the effects of dormant pathogens. Ewald came to believe that slumbering low-grade and long-standing infections were the next frontier for the germ theory of disease. He calls them "the stealth infections."[8]

In 2006, Siobhán M. O'Connor, then assistant director at the US Centers for Disease Control, wrote, "Evidence now confirms that noncommunicable chronic diseases can stem from infectious agents. Furthermore, at least 13 of 39 recently described infectious agents induce chronic syndromes." Later in the same paper, she noted, "Infectious agents likely determine more cancers, immune-mediated syndromes, neurodevelopmental disorders, and other chronic conditions than currently appreciated."[9] Her latter point is easily corroborated. See, for example this passage from Wise Geek, a website which describes itself as offering "clear answers to common questions" and reaches a million unique visitors per month. After defining a chronic disease as one that persists or recurs and usually affects a person for three months or more, it states:

> A chronic disease is generally one that is hereditary or one that is the result of factors such as poor diet and living conditions, using tobacco or other harmful substances, or a sedentary lifestyle. Such a disease is not typically contracted from another person by contagion, because most chronic illnesses are not caused by infection. The term chronic disease commonly applies to conditions that can be treated but not necessarily cured.[10]

A 2010 report from the World Health Organization (WHO) on noncommunicable diseases has a wealth of information about the burden the world faces as a result of chronic illnesses. This authoritative source tells us that they are by far the leading cause of death worldwide. They kill 36 million people annually, a quarter of them under the age of sixty.[11] In 2011, another report from WHO offered detailed profiles of chronic diseases in all the world's countries, from Afghanistan to Zimbabwe.[12] And an accompanying fact sheet states, "Noncommunicable—or chronic—diseases are diseases of long duration and generally slow progression. The four main types of noncommunicable diseases are cardiovascular diseases (like heart attacks and stroke), cancer, chronic respiratory diseases (such as chronic obstructed pulmonary disease and asthma) and diabetes."[13] Ewald published his book about stealth infections in 2000, but the idea that you might "catch" a chronic disease still seems to be novel. Here even the WHO, which elsewhere has acknowledged that liver cancer, stomach cancer, and cervical cancer are the result of pathogens, appears to be equating "chronic" with "noncommunicable."

A chronic infection is not always stealthy. Patients with tuberculosis, for instance, may experience an acute phase at the beginning of their illness, tire easily, feel slightly feverish, and cough frequently. Four to eight weeks after being infected with HIV, many people develop flu-like symptoms such as a sore throat, headache, mild fever, fatigue, muscle and joint pains, swelling of the lymph nodes, rash, and (occasionally) oral ulcers. These symptoms usually last from between one and two weeks. True stealth infections are a subset of the chronic. They arrive unannounced and stay hidden for a long time. A woman might harbor human papillomavirus for decades without being aware of it, before eventually developing cervical abnormalities. Ewald draws our attention to just such surreptitious invaders, believing they may be responsible for a number of cancers, diabetes, arthritis, atherosclerosis, multiple sclerosis, and perhaps even mental illnesses such as autism, schizophrenia, and depression.

The human body contains a vast populace of microbes, including bacteria, fungi, and viruses. There are ten times as many of them as there are somatic cells in the body, up to 100 trillion in an adult (500 times the number of stars in the Milky Way). Each of us hosts thousands of different species of bacteria alone, and we haul around between three and five pounds of them in our gastrointestinal tract. They contain somewhere between 10 and 20 million protein-coding genes—a figure that dwarfs the 23,000 in the human genome. Microorganisms dust the skin and eyes and nestle down in the nose and mouth; the vast majority of bacteria are the gut flora living in the large intestine. Robert Holt, the head of gene sequencing at the BC Cancer Agency, said, "We are basically walking incubators." Walt Whitman wasn't thinking about this phenomenon, but his words from "Song of Myself" are an apt description: "I am large—I contain multitudes." Some of the gut flora perform useful tasks; they help us to digest carbohydrates. Others are thought to be neither helpful nor harmful. But this teeming population is not well understood. According to Holt, the universe of organisms within us "has been largely ignored. The only ones that have percolated to people's awareness are those that have been easily and readily linked to various infections or cancers." In 2008, the US National Institutes of Health launched a five-year Human Microbiome Project with a budget of $157 million to sequence the genomes of the microbes in the human body and elucidate their relationship to human health. It is quite probable that surprising connections to both acute and chronic diseases will emerge.

Pathogens that cause chronic infections are masters of adaptation. They are at home in different kinds of cells and can successfully evade the immune system for many years. Because they adopt a multiplicity of strategies to establish long-term residency in our bodies, they can cause a multiplicity of illnesses too. HIV, for instance, sneaks into immune cells, making it very hard for the system to strike it. Herpes lurks in nerve tissue, which the immune system tends not to target. A hepatitis B–infected liver cell produces about a thousand times as many empty viral shells as full ones. These decoys soak up neutralizing antibodies, leaving large amounts of potent viruses circulating in the blood.[14] Some microbes use molecular mimicry—disguising themselves as their host's cells—to remain inconspicuous. This is thought to be part of the explanation for autoimmune diseases. If the immune system is confused about what is self and what is other, it may attack its own tissues. Some oncoviruses deconstruct themselves and sequester their DNA in their host's cellular genome, beyond reach of the immune system. The danger posed by the flexibility and resilience of these agents is not always appreciated. Ewald writes that pathogens have often been "grievously underestimated."[15] He reminds us that in the past, people who suggested infectious causes for diseases were wrongly dismissed as cranks or worse. Ewald is determined to see that we don't make the same mistake again.

Ever since the Genome Project was concluded in 2000, scientists have ramped up their search for mutations that might be responsible for common chronic diseases. It seems that hardly a month goes by without another announcement—that a "gene for" depression, autism, or obesity has been discovered. (The *New Yorker* spoofed this in a recent cartoon: a wife reading the newspaper turns to her husband and says, "They've found the nebbish gene.") Ewald wants to be sure that in our enthusiasm for genetic explanations, we don't ignore their limitations—especially as a possible account of *common* diseases. He takes his cue from the logic of evolutionary fitness and natural selection. He said, "If an allele [a variant of a gene] is very detrimental, it's going to be weeded out." Ewald credits his colleague, Cochran, for stressing the importance of this: "The idea is kicking around a lot in genetics. It's not new to Greg. But Greg was very forceful in applying it."

Evolutionarily fit individuals produce viable offspring who pass on their genes to the next generation. You can also consider the contribution that an individual makes to the survival and reproduction of other people, siblings and grandchildren, who share some of their genes. The British geneticist J. B. S. Haldane is credited for first noticing the phenomenon. Bill Hamilton called it "inclusive fitness" and proposed that it offers a mechanism for the evolution of altruism.[16] If an allele increases evolutionary fitness, it will become more prevalent in the population. Generally, if it damages those who have it and diminishes their ability to reproduce, it will become less prevalent. Even alleles that reduce fitness by just a small amount gradually dwindle as fewer and fewer copies appear in successive generations. You could say they contain within themselves the seeds of their own destruction. While damaging mutations can crop up spontaneously, they are always rare, and so the harm they do to the total population will be restricted. (Duchenne's muscular dystrophy is one of the most common ailments arising this way, yet it affects fewer than two out of ten thousand people.)

If mutations that impair fitness do sometimes persist, it is only because they have some offsetting benefit. Sickle-cell anemia, a disease which causes red blood cells to change their shape and become curved like a sickle, is probably the most famous example. The cells clump up, don't flow well in small blood vessels, die quickly, and fail to deliver oxygen efficiently. People with the illness are vulnerable to infections and strokes. Before the advent of modern medicine, it was almost always fatal in children. Its effect on their evolutionary fitness was disastrous. Yet the allele responsible for the disease is not rare. How could this be? "You know," said Ewald, "that the only way it could be that common is because it's a genetic disease with a compensating benefit. That idea is what led some people early on to suspect that it was providing protection against malaria." In 1949, at a conference in Italy, J. B. S. Haldane was one of the first to suggest this might be going on.[17] Later, another British researcher, Anthony Allison, showed that while individuals with two copies of the sickle-cell allele developed anemia, people with one copy were more likely to survive malaria.[18] For years, scientists have been trying to understand why this is so. Although it probably doesn't settle the question, research published in 2011 may bring us closer to an answer. People with one copy of the gene almost never have any problems as a result. But the presence of some sickle-cell hemoglobin seems to increase the production of a malaria-combating enzyme.[19] There are other examples. If you have two copies of the mutated CFTR gene, you will develop cystic fibrosis, a deadly disease that attacks the lungs. Having one copy, though, apparently protects you from typhoid.

Ewald calls diseases like sickle-cell anemia "self destructive defenses." They endure because they provide resistance to infection. Neither sickle-cell anemia nor cystic fibrosis would be as common as they are without the lethal infections from which they protect us. If a dangerous pathogen becomes less common, a mutation which helps us to resist it also dwindles. Thus in Africa, where malaria is endemic, one out of five people carry the sickle-cell allele; in the United States, however, only one in twelve African Americans have it. All of this serves to remind us of the critical role that pathogens play. Deleterious genes can cause rare diseases, to be sure. But for them to cause a disease which is not rare, they must offer a benefit—help us combat a microbe, for example. The story of such a disease is also the story of a microorganism which determines its prevalence.

A key consideration for Ewald is that pathogens, unlike damaging mutations, can afflict large numbers of us for indefinite periods of time without providing any offsetting advantages whatsoever. They have been with us from the beginning, when hominid creatures began moving into the African savannah. And when we invented agriculture ten thousand years ago and started living in larger, settled communities, they were there too. In fact, they profited from our invention, as it brought the susceptible hosts closer together, making it easier for them to spread and multiply. They have been with us in peacetime and in war—especially in war. You can almost think of war as our gift to pathogens. In wartime, masses of people often move to places they have never visited before, carrying microbes and introducing them to fresh victims. The combat weakens human beings, rendering their immune systems less effective. War is a feast for pathogens.

As Ewald says, "We are their food."[20] Microbes have their own agenda and when it comes to common diseases are, therefore, prime suspects. Although we evolve in response to microbes, they change and develop better ways of penetrating our immune systems. What Ewald calls "an evolutionary arms race"[21] ensues, but the germs persist. They evolve faster than we do. In the span of one human generation, fifty thousand generations of *E. coli* come and go. Circulating strains of influenza change so rapidly that every year the flu vaccine needs to be updated in order to remain effective. This adaptability gives infectious agents significant firepower and staying power; no wonder some are as old as humanity. Molecular evidence from Peruvian and Egyptian mummies demonstrates that tuberculosis, Chagas disease, smallpox, and polio are thousands of years old.[22] Malaria may be even older. Researchers recently reported that this illness, which now infects 230 million people every year, evolved alongside modern humans and moved with our ancestors as they migrated out of Africa around 60,000 to 80,000 years ago.[23]

Environmental hazards are on Ewald's list of possible causes of disease. He thinks, however, that they are unlikely to be responsible for illnesses that have troubled humanity for a long time. He points out that if we are exposed to non-infectious risks, we will gradually develop defenses in response. Unlike microbes, these factors don't evolve new offensive strategies, so you can anticipate that natural selection would reduce our susceptibility to them. "Skin color is a good example," Ewald said. "If you've got a lot of exposure to UV light over many generations you will develop dark skin color and you're not so prone to cancer." Another illustration is the ability Tibetans have to thrive at high altitudes and low oxygen levels. A 2010 study comparing the genomes of fifty Tibetans and forty Han Chinese found that ethnic Tibetans split off from the Han less than three thousand years ago and since then have rapidly evolved unique genetic adaptations to their punishing mountain home. When people from lower elevations move above about 13,000 feet, where oxygen levels are about 40 percent lower than at sea level, they tire easily, develop headaches, produce babies with lower birth weights, and have a higher infant mortality rate. Tibetans have none of these problems.[24]

Of course, we are still vulnerable to *novel* environmental insults—toxins, the ills of modern civilization. These sometimes act on their own—like Minamata disease, which was first noticed in Japan in 1956. When a chemical factory released methylmercury into a local harbor from 1932 to 1968, more than twelve thousand citizens in Minamata City developed debilitating neurological symptoms. New environmental perils can also aggravate the effect of infections or genetic dispositions. A recent Swedish study showed that smoking, which has been popular among women only since World War II, exacerbates the effect of HPV.[25] Infected women who smoke more than double their risk of developing cervical cancer.

If a disease is old, new toxins or modern lifestyle choices are not going to provide the whole account of it. They may contribute to the contemporary manifestation of the illness, but they won't explain why the disease existed thousands of years ago. Tellingly, many chronic diseases are ancient. In 2011, CT scans of Egyptian mummies dating back to 1981 BC found evidence of hardening of the arteries.[26] The Ebers papyrus, which dates to 1550 BC, contains a description of a disease which could very well be diabetes mellitus; and another Egyptian document, the Edwin Smith papyrus, written between 3000 and 2500 BC, contains an account of breast cancer (and a suggested palliative measure—cauterization). In 2007, a research team found that the mummified remains of a Scythian king who had lived 2,700 years ago in Russia contained evidence of metastasizing prostate cancer.[27] They made the determination based on the microscopic examination of the bone lesions and the presence of PSA (prostate-specific antigen), a marker of prostate cancer. In 2003, a radiologist pushed back the history of cancer even further when he found twenty-nine tumors in the bones of ninety-seven hadrosaurs, or "duck-billed dinosaurs," that lived in the Cretaceous period about 70 million years ago.[28] Thus, Ewald and Cochran write: "When diseases have been common in human populations for many generations and still have a substantial negative impact on fitness, they are likely to have infectious causes."[29]

It's important to remember that evolutionary fitness can persist beyond our reproductive years. Grandparents can help their grandchildren survive. But once people approach advanced old age, a disease which seriously damages them wouldn't have much impact on their descendants. The argument for an infectious cause is less compelling. Ewald said, "Because natural selection acts at younger ages, any characteristic you have as a result of mutations that provides a benefit at a young age but a cost at an older age is going to be favored. It seems almost inevitable that at some age, you're going to have organs that are paying the price for some adaptation that allows them to function earlier. You could apply this to coronary artery disease. If fat storage is useful, there's a price you pay if you have fat storage for a hundred years." Common diseases which hit in old age *could* be caused by infections, but they could also be caused by genes which are passed on from generation to generation. There would be no mechanism for weeding them out. What you might call Ewald's mantra, "Seek the pathogen," is not a methodological directive that applies to all diseases. However, it does add to the range of illnesses for which seeking an infectious agent makes sense.

In their investigations of chronic diseases, scientists have made the most progress finding the microbes linked to cancer. "Right now we know," Ewald said, "that 20 percent of human cancers are caused by infections." Since the early sixties and the discovery of the oncogenic Epstein-Barr virus, the number of malignancies attributed to the action of microbes has steadily increased. "But people's mindsets in medicine haven't quite caught up with that," Ewald observed. He thinks researchers still expect that *future* discoveries will indict genes or environmental mutagens—not pathogens. "Let's keep the viewpoint that is actually scientifically rigorous," he advises. "We don't know at this point what causes the rest of the 80 percent of cancers but infectious causes are a very good candidate because most of those cancers are *associated* with infection."

Even lung cancer, which is generally attributed to smoking, may also involve a virus. Ewald said, "We know that smoking is playing a role—an essential or important exacerbating role. But we also know that nonsmokers get cancer and that a lot of smokers don't get lung cancer." (Studies vary, but worldwide about 10 to 25 percent of lung cancers occur in people who have never smoked;[30] one out of six male smokers and one out of nine female smokers develop lung cancer.[31]) Ewald wondered whether smokers developed lung cancer if they were also infected with JC virus. Discovered in 1971, and given the initials of the person in whom it was found, it can cause a lethal brain disorder in someone whose immune system is compromised. According to Ewald, "the JC virus belongs to a highly oncogenic family [polyomas] and it's found in lung cancers." In other words, it may provide a missing part of the puzzle. But he worries: "Once people get into their head that lung cancers are caused by smoking it closes them off from thinking more broadly about the other possibilities."

MY JAW IS STILL DROPPING ON THIS

Ewald has been described as someone who "likes to think like a pathogen." When I asked him if that was true, he laughed and said, "Of course pathogens don't think." And then he went on to say, "But it's important to be able to look at a problem from every point of view. In medicine we have historically been thinking from the point of view of humans. Our concern is how to help the humans." For Ewald, if you're taking the perspective of a pathogen that causes cancer you should ask *why* it causes the malignancy—how does this help it survive and reproduce better than its competition? "It's important to realize," he said, "that the virus isn't benefiting from the cancer, it is benefiting from *persistence*. Viruses that are transmitted very infrequently would be under very strong selective pressure to be persistent." Earlier, when Ewald was looking at why some microbes are more virulent than others, he discovered that their mode of transmission was a crucial factor. Here again it was influential.

Viruses spread by sexual contact and intimate kissing are under pressure to persist, Ewald noted. In many cases they might have to wait months or even years before their hosts present them with the prospect of infecting another individual. A virus like hepatitis B that passes from mother to child during birth may face even more restricted opportunities. This may help to explain why it makes much of every chance it gets and why in Taiwan, before any vaccines were deployed, the transmission of hepatitis B viruses was so efficient. After spreading to 95 percent of the babies of carrier mothers, the viruses launched asymptomatic infections which allowed them to colonize other infants two, three, or even four decades later. Most of the infected babies seemed perfectly healthy. But they were carriers too, and if they were female and had children, those infants would also be infected. Ludwik Gross suggested in his discussion of vertically transmitted cancers that those who spread such diseases were likely to be "latent carriers." We can see by looking at hepatitis B why this makes sense. If liver cancer hit men and (particularly) women in their child-bearing years or earlier, the pathogen would never have spread so widely.

A virus that establishes a chronic infection initiates changes that over a long period of time may result in cancer. Ewald said, "It just so *happens* that one of the best ways to persist is by breaking the barriers to cancer." Before I met Paul Ewald, he sent me the draft of a book that he and Holly Swain Ewald had written—*Controlling Cancer: A Powerful Plan for Taking On the World's Most Daunting Disease*."[32] In order to grasp why cancer occurs, they look in detail at what HPV does to maintain long-term residence in the cells it infects.

Elizabeth Schwarz opened the door to this understanding in 1984 when she showed that the two genes E6 and E7 are active in cervical cancer cells. The Ewalds explain that these genes inhibit four major cellular defenses the body has against disease. What are those barriers? First, if something is amiss, if a mutation has occurred or a pathogen has attacked, a cell can stop dividing. This prevents copies of the diseased cell from proliferating. Secondly, if the problem cannot be fixed, the cell initiates suicide (known as apoptosis). This is an orderly process that takes place many times a day; in an average adult, between 50 and 70 billion cells self-destruct due to apoptosis. Thirdly, cells normally enforce a cap on the total number of divisions they undergo. If the limit is removed, they can go on indefinitely, like cell lines derived from Henrietta Lacks's tumor. She was thirty-one when she died in 1951. The cell lines grown from her cancer are now much older than she became. Provided with nutrients, they are immortal. Finally, cells usually promote their adherence to nearby cells. When these bonds break down, the cells are free to travel throughout the body and grow in several places. In other words, metastasizing cancer develops. E6 releases proteins that take the brakes off cell division. E7 encourages metastasis.

HPV's ability to endure has helped it triumph during the evolutionary arms race. In the US, it is the most widespread sexually transmitted infection. A 2007 study showed that almost 50 percent of sexually active American women between the ages of twenty and twenty-four have HPV.[33] And men are not immune. According to a 2011 study of adult men from eighteen to seventy in Brazil, Mexico, and the United States, half had some form of the virus.[34] While women's chance of contracting HPV declines as they grow older, men appear to be at high risk of acquiring new HPV infections throughout their lives. The likelihood of developing a malignancy even from high-risk HPVs is very low.[35] Less than 2 percent of women who have these viruses develop cervical cancer. Men who have them can get anal, penile, head, and neck cancers, but the probability of such outcomes is also small. Nevertheless, because the infection is so common, the total number of cases is significant; globally, more than a quarter of a million women die every year from cervical cancer.

From the virus's "point of view," all that is necessary is to persist and produce copies of its own genome. Cancer is irrelevant; it doesn't serve the virus's "interests." But in effect, its manipulations clear the decks for a malignancy. Cells carrying the viral genome can reproduce indefinitely without limit; even though they are defective, they no longer obey signals to self-destruct. Moreover, these cells can start new colonies throughout the host's body.

All of this creates the conditions necessary for the wild reproduction that we know as cancer, but it is not sufficient to tip the balance. As the Ewalds explain, E6 and E7 get the cells dividing, but not so much that they pose a lethal threat to the person. However, at some point there is a major transformation. The infected cells begin replicating in such a way that they are a serious menace. In the case of HPV, the integration of its genes into the genome of the host cell is part of that dangerous transformation. But it is not the whole story. Additional factors—not completely understood yet—also play a supporting role. It is important to realize that unless HPV gets there first, those elements won't create a malignancy; the cancer will not begin. That's why, even though we don't have a full account of how cervical cancer arises, we still know enough to intervene successfully.

According to Ewald, other cancer-causing viruses compromise the same barriers HPV sabotages. He told me that bacteria apparently behave in a similar fashion. "Look at *Helicobacter pylori*. It knocks out some of the same barriers, which is a bit surprising because viruses *have* to do that for them to be able to persist long-term in the cells and bacteria wouldn't necessarily have to do that. They could have a lot of other tricks up their sleeve for persistence." Ewald's study of the role that HPV plays in cancer is leading him toward a radical inference. He told me, "We can't say this conclusively, but it sure looks like it's extremely difficult to get cancer *without* infection." Ewald explained that while some environmental agents might "ratchet up" the mutation rate, that in itself would not necessarily compromise the four specific and significant defenses the body has against cancer. All it might do is cause mutations that are negative for the cells' viability. In other words, in order to get cancer a little sleight of hand is required. Ewald said, "You've got to get the mutations that lead to it without getting the vastly more numerous mutations that make cells non-functional."

YOU HAVE TO HAVE A GOOD CONCEPTUAL STRUCTURE

Ewald is embarking on an ambitious project—the subject of an upcoming book. He is aiming to describe nothing less than a unified theory of cancer—a daunting goal. He said, "There's always this argument about the right way to do science. Going back to Descartes and Harvey, and some of the early medical scientists, there's been this tension between people who think that if you just get the evidence in an objective way, the truth will emerge, and the scientists who say we need to come up with a hypothesis." I hear in this an echo of Pasteur, who said, "Theory alone can bring forth and develop the spirit of invention." Ewald worries about investigators who plow ahead with no overarching picture of where they are going and who modestly aim "to get this small piece of the puzzle." He explained:

> You've got to get somebody saying, "Wait a minute, we have 10 million pieces of the puzzle. Which pieces aren't really relevant and which are?" When we talk about cancer, it is clear we're in the midst of a crisis. Every day there are 250 papers on cancer published. Just go to PubMed [the US National Library of Medicine's free database] and it's staggering to think you can never master all of this. To me the way that we're going to make progress is to have organizing principles tell us where the critical bits of information are. You have to have a good conceptual structure. That's where natural selection comes in, the conceptual structure for studying living things. There's nothing else that is as powerful an explanation of why everything is the way it is.

We had been conversing for hours. At the end of our interview, Ewald told me stories about the people who had gone before him—Charles Darwin, J. B. S. Haldane, George Williams. He told me about Bill Hamilton, a great theorist and a man "who was always doing dangerous things." Ewald said, "He was in Rwanda in the middle of the furor, collecting insects when he was arrested. When he was asked, 'What are you doing' he said, 'I'm collecting insects—these beetles I'm interested in.'" He was released when his colleagues at Oxford vouched for him, saying that he really was collecting beetles and wasn't a spy. Hamilton was determined to understand the etiology of AIDS. That was why he flew to Africa in 2000 and began collecting chimpanzee scat to see whether it contained any viruses ancestral to HIV. He contracted malaria and took an aspirin for pain. For some reason, it caused a hemorrhage. Perhaps because he was also suffering from ulcers, he never recovered from it. Once again I was reminded of the commitment scientists have to their subjects. The truths they find are often hard-won.

When it was time for lunch, Paul Ewald's wife, Holly, joined us and we went to the Mayan Café. It was probably Louisville's most interesting restaurant, and for the first time, I tasted a mole sauce. Afterward, Paul drove me to the airport, and I headed back to rainy Vancouver. On the flight, I began thinking about stealth infections. I found the idea that I might be harboring an untold number of these unsettling. I knew it was unlikely that anything untoward might happen, but there was still a chance of it. It made me feel a little like a walking time bomb. On the other hand, I reflected, as we discover more about these pathogens, we will probably learn how to prevent them with vaccines, or treat them with antibiotics and antivirals. We won't be unwittingly perpetuating a silent epidemic like the hepatitis B contagion Beasley discovered in Taiwan. The long incubation period of stealth infections dramatically increases the possibility for intervention and prevention. I thought about cervical cancer. It was always the poster child for early intervention. The PAP smear enabled physicians to discover pre-cancerous lesions, treat those, and forestall a full-blown cancer. Now, of course, we have a vaccine. But even for those women who have not been vaccinated, there is hope. We should be able to push intervention back several steps. By testing a woman for HPV, we might be able to stop the stealth infection in its tracks *decades before* those telltale lesions occur. The strategies pathogens developed to persist and maximize their chances of spreading to other hosts are their strength—and their Achilles heel.

The idea that pathogens can cause cancer was given much publicity recently when Barry Marshall, Robin Warren, and Harald zur Hausen all received Nobel Prizes for their work. But as Ewald pointed out to me, much more work is required. "What we need are studies that look for pathogens that are *associated* with cancer, that we haven't discovered yet, or ones that test whether the associations we have discovered are causal." In fact, new biochemical techniques are making that search for associations much easier. I will turn to that subject in my last chapter.

6

GENE HUNTERS

Our discovery was greeted with scorn, derision.

—Patrick Moore

In mid-December 1994, at a Columbia University news conference, a husband and wife team, Yuan Chang and Patrick Moore, stood in front of an assembly of reporters. They had something to announce—a finding that was being published in *Science* magazine.[1] Chang was an assistant professor of pathology at Columbia who had arrived in New York just about two years before, in January 1993. She'd started the research project which culminated in the press conference with a modest grant of $15,000 from the Columbia University Pathology Department. It was barely enough money to buy the chemicals she needed for the research, but at least it allowed her to begin. Moore, like Chang, was a physician, and also a recent arrival in New York. Before coming, he'd been working for the CDC in Nigeria, where he'd stickhandled an outbreak of hemorrhagic fever. He was also seconded to refugee camps in Somalia—just before the famous Black Hawk Down incident where Somali militia shot down an American helicopter. Moore decided he was allergic to lead—fast-moving lead—and moved back to the United States. His first job on his return home was as deputy commissioner at the New York City Department of Health. He left it in March 1994 to work full time with Chang. Since their results were so promising, Columbia University hired him as an assistant professor of public health.

Suddenly the two scientists were facing the scrutiny of the world. *Newsday*'s Laurie Garrett, a reporter and recent author of a book about

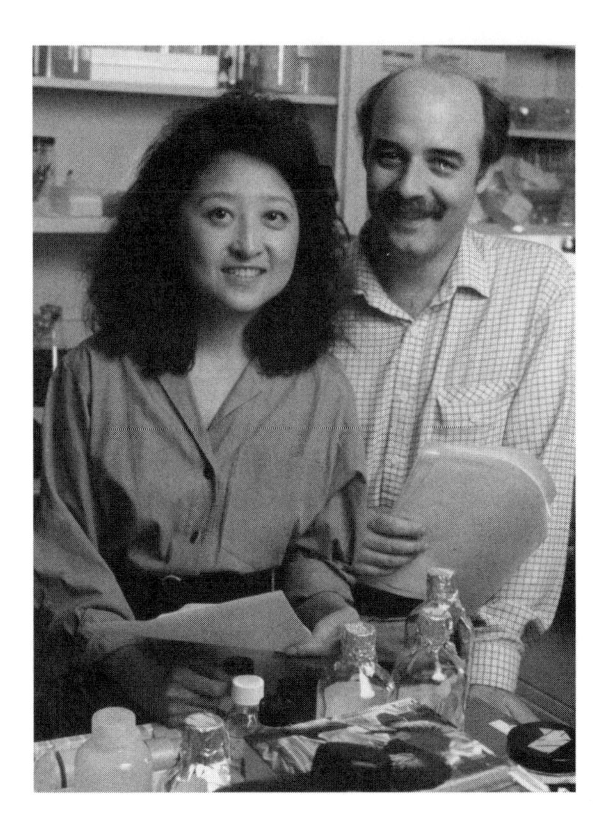

Figure 6.1. Patrick Moore and Yuan Chang in 1995. Photo courtesy of Columbia University

infectious diseases, had come, as well as the *Wall Street Journal*'s senior science writer, Jerry Bishop. Lawrence Altman, the physician journalist from the *New York Times*, was also there. The headline of his subsequent story, "Going Off the Beaten Path to Track Down Clues about AIDS,"[2] hinted at how unusual all this was. Chang and Moore had used a novel technique to find a virus. Newcomers to the field, they'd tackled a problem that had baffled much more experienced and distinguished researchers. If they were right about their observations, these "upstarts" had pulled off quite a coup.

Science not only published Moore and Chang's research paper. It also published an article about it. The author, Jon Cohen, interviewed a number of experts who had different views. Bernard Roizman (who had dismissed Harald zur Hausen's findings in 1972) was enthusiastic. He said, "I think it's real." Harold Jaffe, head of the HIV/AIDS division at the CDC, said, "I think it is a very good candidate." But Elliott Kieff, director of infectious diseases at Boston's Brigham & Womens' Hospital, warned, "It may turn out to be just a passenger." Robert Gallo, a distinguished virologist who contributed much to the discovery that HIV caused AIDS, was cautious. Though he praised Chang and Moore's paper for being "careful," he said, "I have major questions."[3]

The mystery that Chang and Moore tried to solve concerned the cause of the recent American outbreak of Kaposi's sarcoma (KS) which afflicted some AIDS patients. The disease caused small purplish skin cancers and was often fatal. It was not a new illness. In 1872, Moritz Kaposi, a Hungarian physician in Vienna, had seen a group of patients with these lesions and identified their condition as a malignancy. For a long time, it was rare. American physicians would occasionally find it in elderly Jewish or African patients. But in the early 1980s an unusually large number of young men began visiting their physicians to complain of those same lesions. Why was this skin disease that had previously afflicted just a few elderly men showing up in a significant population of young Americans? It turned out that the patients who were visiting their doctors about the disturbing skin eruptions had AIDS. Their lesions were the visible sign of a devastating epidemic—the pox of the disease. Did that mean that HIV, which caused AIDS, also caused Kaposi's sarcoma?

In 1987, Harald Jaffe and Valerie Beral, a professor from Oxford University and visiting scientist at the CDC, teamed up to find out. They discovered that in the US, Kaposi's sarcoma was twenty thousand times more common in persons with AIDS than in the general population. Still AIDS alone did not seem to explain the illness. At that time, gay or bisexual men were at risk for developing AIDS, but hemophiliacs were too. They got it from blood transfusions. Beral and Jaffe discovered that people with AIDS were twenty times more likely to develop Kaposi's sarcoma if they were gay or bisexual than if they were hemophiliacs. Yet both groups suffered equally from other symptoms of AIDS. Why were gay men more likely to develop this secondary illness? Some suggested it was the nitrate inhalers, the "poppers" that gay men often used, but others disputed that association. Jaffe and Beral proposed that the sarcoma was transmitted by an unidentified infectious agent through sexual contact, but not blood transfusions.[4] The sarcoma seemed to be caused by the intersection of AIDS, which depressed the immune system, *and* something else which took advantage of a patient's weakened state. What was it?

Many virologists tried hard to solve the puzzle. They had already proffered twenty candidate germs as possible causes for the deadly sarcoma. None of the suggestions panned out. However, Chang and Moore had a different approach, a new way of finding viruses, or, to be more specific, virus DNA, and they thought they could succeed where so many others had not.

WOULDN'T IT BE NICE IF WE COULD USE GENETIC TECHNIQUE TO IDENTIFY PATHOGENS?

I spoke to Patrick Moore a couple of times on the phone, and we had a lively email exchange as well. He is now the director of the Cancer Virology Program at the University of Pittsburgh Cancer Institute, and Yuan Chang is a professor of pathology there. Moore told me that he was born in October 1956 in Utah. His mother was a Christian Scientist, his father a Mormon. "So I became a doctor who drank and smoked—naturally," he said. He remembered his parents as "extremely tolerant, amazing people." They encouraged him to get interested in science "beyond what was offered in school, and beyond getting good grades." Like Harald zur Hausen and Barry Marshall, Moore read scientific biographies as a child. In the fourth grade, Marie Curie became his heroine (and remained so for about five years). "I did pretty well in elementary school—not outstanding, though—but I was miserable in high school. I dropped out in the eleventh grade. I still don't have my high school diploma. I'll have to go back and get it, or else I'll keep getting lousy jobs like this one!" he said, laughing. Moore took a college entrance exam and did extremely well. He was accepted at a community college in Rockspring, Wyoming, and then transferred to Westminster College in Salt Lake City, where he completed a bachelor's of science in chemistry and biology. He said, "Though I didn't go to a big Ivy League School, I wound up in a place that best suited me."

Moore went on to get a masters in science from Stanford and then entered medical school at the University of Utah. He said that Yuan took "the exact opposite course from me." Born in Taipei, Taiwan, in

November 1959, she moved to the United States as a young girl and grew up in Salt Lake City. Moore said, "She was a very good student in junior high school and high school, went to Wellesley [a select liberal arts college for women in Massachusetts], and then transferred to Stanford. Yuan came back to Utah for medical school." This is where Moore and Chang met, but for several years, they were hardly ever in the same city. Ambitious, and eager to learn as much as possible, they both chalked up a dizzying array of experiences.

Moore worked in Ghana and Liberia and did an internship in Montreal, hoping to learn some French along the way. "Unfortunately," he said, "I picked the Jewish General Hospital, so I learned more Yiddish than French, which is okay, but it doesn't help in Francophone Africa." After his internship, he joined the CDC's Epidemic Investigation Service (EIS)—the same organization that sent Palmer Beasley to Bolivia. Moore investigated pneumococcal meningitis epidemics and squeezed in a masters in public health (on AIDS prevention). He worked for the CDC as an epidemiologist at Fort Collins in Colorado, where he studied viruses transmitted by spiders. Then the CDC sent him to Nigeria, where he found himself in the middle of a serious outbreak. He said, "People were bleeding out of their ears and their eyes. We had no idea whether it was Lhasa or Ebola. One possibility was that it was yellow fever. If it was, we had an excellent vaccine that was made in the 1920s. But we could not figure it out at first; the seriological tests didn't respond the way that we anticipated. I began thinking, 'Wouldn't it be nice if we could use genetic techniques to identify pathogens?'"

Moore and Chang married in 1989, but often lived apart. Chang did a fellowship in pathology at the University of California in San Francisco, and then did another fellowship in a subspecialty, neuropathology, at Stanford. As part of her training she also learned molecular biology techniques and became highly skilled at using them. When Chang was offered a position as an associate professor of pathology at Columbia University, she moved to New York in 1993. At that time, she was interested in tracking down the genes responsible for brain cancer. Moore joined Chang in New York and got a job at the Department of Health. He was still thinking about the idea he'd had during the yellow fever epidemic in Nigeria—about how useful it might be to have efficient techniques for the genetic identification of pathogens. He considered it from time to time and followed the literature that was developing on the subject.

THE ENTIRE FIELD WAS COMPLETELY DISGUSTED AND BURNED OUT

When Moore read a paper by Michael Wigler, who ran a lab in Cold Spring Harbour, New York,[5] it abruptly changed the direction of his career and Yuan's. The paper explained how you could compare two complex genomes and isolate the genes that were different between the two samples. This, it said, "holds promise for the discovery of infectious agents and probes useful for genetic studies." Wigler called the technique representational difference analysis or RDA. No one had actually used it to find an unknown pathogen, but Moore, like Wigler, saw its potential. He asked himself, "Could *we* use that to molecularly identify agents in an outbreak?" Moore showed Yuan the paper. She was also intrigued. So they had a method, but where should they apply it? It wasn't hard for Moore to come up with a proposal—he thought they should look at the big question of the day. Could they find the infectious agent that caused Kaposi's sarcoma? By the time Moore got interested in the problem, he said, "the entire field was completely disgusted and burned out by the science that had been repeatedly shown to be not valid." Moore and Chang decided to give it a go anyway.

Because Chang was a pathologist, she was also part of New York's autopsy service. So when a young Hispanic man who had AIDS and KS died, she was called in to help with the autopsy. Moore said, "After this person came into autopsy, no more autopsies were done on AIDS patients for two years—because of fear of infecting the pathologist and because they thought they couldn't learn anything from it. We got lucky, it turns out. We were in the right place at the right time." After the KS lesions and some nearby healthy tissues were carefully removed from the patient, Chang compared the genetic profiles of the two samples. She "subtracted" the profile of the healthy sample from that of the diseased tissue. Leftover sequences might very well be those of an invading pathogen. Moore said, "It doesn't sound difficult, but it is a tedious experiment to do correctly. It's easy to get contamination. It wasn't a simple thing." Chang worked on the problem in the evenings after completing her other tasks. When she started the project, Moore was still at the New York Health Department. He joined Chang at the lab after his day's work was over. He'd catch the number nine train for Columbia and stay from 7 p.m. to "whenever."

In just five weeks, Chang found an important clue—two viral DNA fragments of interest. She didn't have a whole microbe, mind you, just a piece of one. "It isn't traditional virology," said Moore. "We don't hunt for viruses, we hunt for genes." Chang had isolated less than 1 percent of the total viral genome. Nevertheless, it was enough so that they could begin asking whether they had a fragment that was associated with Kaposi's sarcomas.

Was the sequence present in Kaposi's sarcomas and absent from other tissues? Moore and Chang collaborated with a colleague at Columbia, Ethyl Cesarman, who was interested in lymphomas and had a variety of tissue samples stored. Using the same hybridization techniques that zur Hausen had employed a decade before, they tested some of Cesarman's samples in a randomized fashion. There was good news. The Kaposi's sarcomas they tested were positive for their viral sequences. But there seemed to be bad news too. As controls, they were using lymphoma tumors. Almost all were negative—except for one. Moore was devastated by the news. He thought, "This is so much work and we're running out of money. If this DNA really belongs to a new virus that causes Kaposi's sarcoma, it's got to be something that's specific to KS, because lymphomas don't have the same epidemiology." When he spoke to Cesarman about it, though, she said the one positive control was a rare lymphoma. Its epidemiology was not well understood, so the news wasn't really so bad after all. (In fact, later the virus Chang had discovered was shown to cause the unusual lymphoma.)

The association between the virus fragments and Karposi's sarcoma was beginning to stand up. This meant Moore and Chang could move on to other questions. What kind of virus had they discovered? At the time, computer algorithms were being established to help investigators match a fragment of interest with identified genetic sequences of viruses stored in databases. Moore had a McIntosh Classic, a little box with a video monitor inside a computer. He had about twenty floppy disks which contained the entire viral database of the day. He put the disks into the computer and, one by one, compared what was on the disks with the viral fragments he had. Then a colleague, Frank Lee, got him access to a new program called the Basic Local Alignment Search Tool—or BLAST alignment. This speeded up the process. Moore learned that the virus fragments Chang had discovered were similar to those of herpesvirus saimeri—a microbe that infects squirrel monkeys. It was, however, different enough that it was probably new. It came to be known as KSHV—for Kaposi's sarcoma–associated herpesvirus.

It was the first time anyone had used the RDA technique to detect an unknown pathogen. In retrospect, you could see why the other research had failed. It had aimed to find a known microbe in KS tumors. However, the pathogen was new. When zur Hausen used genetic probes to discover HPV 16 and 18, he had some idea of what he was looking for. But you could use RDA even if you did not. That made it an ideal technique for detecting what was truly novel.

When Moore and Chang were satisfied they had discovered something significant, they sent off a report to *Science*. A couple of months after it was published, the journal published another paper indicating that several labs around the world were getting similar results. Then the National Cancer Institute (NCI) decided the subject was interesting enough to convene a conference—the first ever—on AIDS-related Kaposi's sarcoma.

Researchers came to NCI headquarters in Bethesda, Maryland, on June 5 and 6, 1995, to learn and debate the new findings. The meeting was rancorous. Jon Cohen from *Science* was there and wrote, "Gallo's withering critique of KSHV packed a punch. If the fragment were part of a virus which caused KS, Gallo said, 'This would be the most unorthodox virus in nature.'"[6] Since the fragment seemed to be part of a herpesvirus, he expected that it would behave like other herpesviruses, which were known to spread widely through the population. But AIDS-KS was found only among gay men, so how could a common virus be its cause? Recalling this, Patrick Moore explained, "Virologists came up with some postulates about how these viruses should behave. One of them was that a herpesvirus is ubiquitous. Everyone should be infected with it." That was true of many of the herpesviruses that had been discovered up until then, for instance, the ones causing cold sores (herpes simplex type 1), chicken pox (varicella-zoster virus), and mononucleosis (Epstein-Barr virus). Moore said the idea was, "If you find a new herpesvirus, it's got to be universal, it's got to be ubiquitous. But if everybody is infected, then how can you explain the epidemiology that just gay men are susceptible?"

Gallo also argued that HIV itself might play a central role in Kaposi's sarcoma—despite the confounding epidemiology. People who had HIV were much more likely to get KS if they were gay than if they were hemophiliacs. Equally puzzling was the fact that some people developed the illness without having HIV at all. These people were at risk because their immune systems were depressed—they had organ transplants and were taking immunosuppressant drugs or were very elderly.

As the investigators at the Bethesda conference pushed and pulled at the data, the picture emerging seemed confusing. Some researchers reported failing to find the new virus where they thought it should be. Others found it in all sorts of skin lesions—basal and squamous cell carcinomas, premalignant keratoses, common warts. Robert Biggar, an NCI epidemiologist, said sarcastically, "Suddenly, we've found the cause of all cancers."[7] Moore told me, "Our discovery was greeted with scorn, derision." Nevertheless, Chang stood her ground in the furor. She said simply, "It's clear that there is a new herpesvirus and that it's associated with KS."

To silence their critics, Moore and Chang needed to demonstrate that the association between KSHV and Kaposi's sarcoma was causal. Koch's postulates were still considered the gold standard for such a demonstration. But as we have seen, they were often difficult to use in the field of tumor virology. Fortunately, since Koch, a British statistician named Bradford Hill had developed a set of criteria in order to establish a causal link between smoking and lung cancer. These criteria had a more general application, and Moore used them for guidance. Moore said, "The first two years were spent trying to nail down Hill's criteria." Fulfilling two of them was especially important in building the case against KSHV. Moore had to show that it was strongly associated with KS. "The answer was yes. Virtually 100 percent of KS lesions are positive for the virus within the margins of misdiagnosis and bad techniques. It looked like virtually all KS has this virus in it. This was true in different settings, different countries, in different laboratories, and most importantly, among different types of Kaposi's sarcoma: that which occurs in AIDS patients, among the elderly, and even in a very severe form that occurs in Africa." Secondly, Moore needed to demonstrate that exposure to KSHV occurred *before* the onset of KS. This would allay any suspicion that Kaposi's sarcoma came first and created conditions that were favorable for the virus, which arrived later. For help with this, Moore collaborated with Lawrence Kingsley at the University of Pittsburgh and Dr. Shou-Jiang Gao from the school of public health at Columbia University.

Kingsley, an epidemiologist, was an investigator on the Multicenter AIDS Cohort Study with sites in Los Angeles, Chicago, Baltimore, and Pittsburgh. He had been collecting blood samples from primarily gay and bisexual men. Some of them were HIV positive, a few went on to develop AIDS, and a fraction of those went on to develop KS. Because the serum collection stretched back to the early eighties, it essentially allowed Moore to go back in time. He said the first task was to develop a blood test to reliably indicate whether patients had been exposed to KSHV. Once that was available, you could check to see which patients developed Kaposi's sarcoma. It so happened that 80 percent of the patients with KS were infected with the microbe *before* they developed the lesions. Moore said, "Within the boundaries of the test, which was only 80 percent sensitive, yes, everybody was infected and then they were developing KS."[8] You could accurately predict that if patients with AIDS also became infected with KSHV, they were very likely to go on to develop the skin cancer. At the time, Moore said, "This is essentially the last nail in the coffin for proving causality. In my mind there is no question that KSHV causes KS."[9]

The study also disposed of an old red herring. While it was true that people generally became infected with most other herpesviruses during their childhoods, Moore could show that this was definitely not true of KSHV. It was not a ubiquitous infection. The idea that all herpesviruses behaved the same way reminded me of what Robin Warren called "a sort of known fact," something generally believed, but not supported by evidence. Most of us have some assumptions like this; it's not surprising that scientists do too.

In 2009, the International Agency for Research on Cancer (IARC) examined KS in a monograph and concluded, "There is *sufficient evidence* in humans for the carcinogenicity of KSHV."[10]

When I asked Moore if we know how KSHV caused cancer, he said that unlike the high-risk forms of human papilloma virus, its DNA doesn't become integrated into the host's cellular genome. Nevertheless, it targets many of the same proteins that HPV does. It drives the human cells to proliferate and prevents them from killing themselves. It turns off the cells' "suicide switch." Though KSHV's story is not known in such detail as HPV's, it is clear that two elements come into play. The human cells' tumor suppressor proteins are deactivated, and the host's immune system is generally under stress. Moore emphasized that cancer is a dead-end for viruses that affect humans. If the host dies, so does the virus. Moreover, oncogenic viruses aren't normally transmitted from tumors. Moore said, "You don't commonly catch HPV from a woman who has cervical cancer. You catch it from someone who is asymptomatically infected. You don't catch KSHV from people who have KS; it's from people who are asymptomatically affected."

By establishing a long-standing infection, viruses maximize their chances to move on to new people. But once a tumor appears, the virus has usually lost its ability to infect others. Moore said, "The virus is not replicating." This helps to explain one of the obstacles which had long bedeviled tumor virologists. The pathogens aren't reproducing in the cancer tissues; they aren't likely to multiply in the lab either. Moore said, "You can't culture it." As Moore was telling me all of this, I thought it was paradoxical that cancer, which is not a good outcome for us, is not a good outcome for the virus either. But then I remembered what Paul Ewald had told me about evolutionary trade-offs. Cancer is the price some viruses pay to establish a persistent infection.

Kaposi's sarcoma was once a rare disease which the AIDS epidemic thrust into the limelight. Recently, in the United States, the availability of good antiretroviral therapy has managed to reduce its incidence. The therapy slows down the progress of HIV and prevents the damage to a person's immune system. Thus, people infected with HIV are better able to resist opportunistic pathogens such as KSHV. However, in Africa, where antiretroviral therapy is not so readily available, Kaposi's sarcoma is now the second-most common cancer among males and the third-most common among women.[11] A vaccine would certainly help. But, Moore said, "Nobody has done anything on KS even though we know so much about it. At least from a scientific perspective, we know precisely what needs to be done to try to target the virus in this tumor."

Moore and Chang continued to look at cancers that occurred more frequently in patients whose immune systems were depressed, reasoning that, like KS, these were likely to have an infectious origin. Merkel cell carcinoma, a lethal skin cancer often appearing as a flesh-colored or bluish-red nodule on the face, head, or neck, was one of these. "It smelled like it would have an infectious etiology," said Moore. While Moore and Chang developed an interest in Merkel cell carcinoma, they also began wondering whether they could improve on the techniques they had used earlier. Moore explained, "We know that less than 3 percent of coding sequences are for genes. You have a huge amount of DNA that is not coding. Also, when we were looking for viral DNA in the tumor DNA, it turned out the viral DNA was less than 1 out of 3 million base pairs. The fact that we found representational KSHV was spectacularly lucky." (One of the reasons for their success was probably that the Hispanic man who furnished the original sample had an inordinately high viral load.)

Was there a more reliable and efficient way of finding viruses? Moore and Chang believed there was. If a virus causes a malignancy, its genes are producing something, probably a protein, that is getting cells to behave like a cancer. Since RNA is actively involved in the expression of proteins, one way of narrowing down the search is to work with RNA; that way you are dealing with the smaller number of sequences directly related to genes. RNA lends itself to the same kind of analysis that Chang and Moore had already performed with DNA. If you sequence the RNA from a tumor, you can subtract the human RNA from it and, if all goes well, what is left over might very well be viral RNA. To look for pathogens in Merkel cell carcinomas, Moore and Chang decided to develop an approach along these lines. They dubbed it Digital Transcriptome Subtraction. For five years, they collected Merkel cell tumors and recruited a gifted graduate student, Huichen Feng, to help with the investigation. Feng set to work; he subtracted the human RNA from the tumor RNA and sent the difference off for sequencing. Said Moore, "Within twenty-four hours of getting the results back, we knew we had a candidate that could be causing this cancer."

Chang and Moore called the pathogen Merkel cell virus (MCV). It was a member of the polyoma virus family which Ludwik Gross had discovered. The family got its name from its ability to cause cancer in various kinds of tissues. Since polyoma viruses caused cancer in animals, scientists had suspected that some of them might be doing the same in people, but so far, nothing had been pinned on them. Unlike the virus responsible for Kaposi's sarcoma, this one was a common, perhaps even universal infection in older children and adults. It was a classic stealth infection that could exist for years without producing any symptoms. In fact, unless the host's immune system became compromised, it might not reveal any sign of itself whatsoever.

MCV was similar to the human papillomavirus, and so Moore borrowed some molecular methods from Harald zur Hausen to show that its relationship with Merkel cell cancer was causal. Moore discovered that like HPV, MCV insinuated itself into the host's cellular genome. And like Elizabeth Schwarz, who had investigated HPV, he was interested in the point at which the sequences of viral and human genes met. Schwarz had wanted to know where the *virus*'s circular genome opened, in order to understand which of its genes survived integration and which did not. Moore was also interested in this junction, but he had a different question in mind. He wanted to know where the *human* genome opened up to accept the viral sequence. He reasoned that if the viral DNA was always "pasted" into the human genome at the same location, this would show that the cells were clonal. They came from the same mother cell. That meant that the integration happened only once—before the cell became a cancer. The human genome with the inserted viral segment replicated itself and the viral DNA was always in the same spot. Moore said, "This would be very strong evidence that the virus was at the scene of the crime when the crime was committed." If, on the other hand, the integration happened at different places along the human genome, this would indicate the cells weren't clonal. The viral genes might be Johnny-come-latelies that arrived after the cell was transformed into a cancer. What did the research show? Two important observations emerged. The integration point was different in the tumors from different individuals. However, within a tumor, the integration spot was always the same. Furthermore, different tumors within the same person had the same integration region as well. Not surprisingly, tumors that formed as a result of metastasis derived from the same mother cell. The tumor cells were clonal; MCV was a cancer-causing virus, not a benign passenger.[12]

Another vital piece of evidence came from a "knockout" experiment. MCV has a major oncogene called the T-antigen gene (or tumor-antigen gene). Massa Shuda, one of Moore and Chang's postdocs, discovered that it expresses a protein called survivin which promotes cell division and prevents cells from committing suicide. But the gene can be rendered inactive. The single-stranded messenger RNA which carries the gene's instructions for making survivin can be silenced. When it is bound to another single strand of RNA called a short hairpin RNA, the message is blocked. (The interfering fragment is named for its shape—the sharp turn it takes.) If the T-antigen gene is inactive, the Merkel cell tumors stop growing—evidence that it helps to cause the malignancy. Moore said, "They are absolutely dependent on the expression of the viral oncogene in order to survive."

This reminded me of von Knebel Doeberitz's experiment with antisense RNA. I remembered that while he had been able to stop tumor growth in the lab, unfortunately he hadn't been able to duplicate those results in women with cervical cancer. So I asked Moore if a treatment might be possible based on his finding. "I'm so glad you asked," he said, laughing.

> There is a company that is making a small molecule, an inhibitor of survivin. We've now got mouse studies that show that this is potent in inhibiting the tumor. It doesn't eliminate it, at least under the conditions we've tried. But it stops the tumor from growing. All of these remarkable developments have happened in just four years. Prior to 2008, Merkel cell carcinoma was the most deadly skin cancer. It had a very unclear pathology. It had a completely mysterious origin, poorly defined therapies, none of which were particularly good. In the four years since then, we've discovered the cause of this cancer. We have developed tests to be able to detect it in patient tissues, and now we have a rational molecular target that is based on this virus. At least in mice, it seems to be extremely effective in retarding the growth of this tumor. And so that's now going into clinical trials to see if it works.

These new techniques are remarkably efficient, which makes them ideal for virus trolling. There are about a thousand viruses known to infect humans. But there is a world of unknown viruses, perhaps as many as ten thousand, which invade us over the course of our lives. We have no idea what they are doing. But a method like Moore's which allows us to quickly scan for dangerous pathogens could be an invaluable aid. Who knows what we may yet discover?

The IARC recently concluded that Merkel cell virus was probably a cause of cancer in humans. (As of this writing, a monograph about this is being prepared for publication.)[13] Moore said, "We can develop very important treatments and diagnostics for cancer that never were possible before. It's not just some empty intellectual exercise."

THAT ACCELERATED THINGS GREATLY

In 2011, two teams of researchers found a bacterium that may be at the root of colon cancer—thus reminding us that the story of cancer and infections is not just about viruses. It could be that *H. pylori* has partners in crime. Robert Holt, head of sequencing at the British Columbia Cancer Agency Genome Centre, led one group, and Matthew Meyerson, a professor of pathology at Harvard Medical School, directed the second. Holt lives near me in North Vancouver. Since I had been talking to researchers around the world, all the way from Perth in Western Australia to northern Canada, I was pleasantly surprised to find someone in my own backyard. Holt told me he was always interested in science; it was his favorite subject in school. "I liked to tinker with things. I would be working on my tricycle, taking off nuts and bolts when I was three years old. I disassembled all my mother's kitchen appliances. I like to find out how things work."

Holt recognized that one way of finding a cancer-causing pathogen was to troll for it as Moore and Chang had done—by comparing the genomes of healthy and diseased tissue. He said, "The concept has been around for awhile, but only in the last few years have the sequencing costs dropped enough to make it feasible." He thought it made sense to look for a bacterium that caused colon cancer because the colon is continually exposed to such a huge diversity of them.

Holt started with a pilot study and eleven patients. In Victoria, British Columbia, the BC Cancer Agency keeps a Biobank of frozen tumors and matched normal tissue from many different types of cancer. It obtains the tissues from patients who have had surgeries and biopsies and who have consented to their use in research. Holt said, "That accelerated things greatly. In a lot of these studies, a substantial amount of time can be spent just acquiring the relevant samples." In order to narrow down his search, Holt started with RNA rather than DNA—as Moore and Chang did in their Merkel cell carcinoma research. When he compared the RNA from the tumor with the RNA from the healthy tissue, he saw that both contained the genomes of about one thousand bacteria. This was normal; he'd expected to find about as many microbes. What he didn't expect, though, was to see that one bacterium was far more common in the cancers than in the normal tissues. This was *Fusobacterium nucleatum*, a long, thin, foul-smelling bacterium. Holt knew this was mostly an oral pathogen; it liked to live in dental plaque, where it caused gum disease. So what was it doing in the gut? Recently scientists had discovered that *F. nucleatum* didn't just live in the mouth. In January 2011, a group of German investigators established that it was responsible for a majority of acute appendicitis cases too.[14] The microbe's theater of operations included internal organs. Furthermore, like another infamous gut bacteria, *H. pylori*, *F. nucleatum* could penetrate epithelial cells and cause inflammation. This just heightened Holt's suspicions; inflammation is already associated with colon cancer. "If *Fusobacterium nucleatum* were a common benign bacterium, we wouldn't have taken much interest in it. But the fact that it was known to cause disease made the case sufficiently compelling to continue the research." Holt decided to investigate a larger sample of ninety-nine people. He found that *F. nucleatum* was 415 times more common in the tumors than in the normal tissue. In addition, he noticed that people with higher bacteria counts were more likely to have regional lymph node metastasis—indicating a more serious disease. Holt said, "That verified that there was a strong tumor association." His finding was published in *Genome Research*, in October of 2011.[15] A study by Matt Myerson appeared in the same issue. He had also identified the bacterium as a possible culprit, using DNA rather than RNA. The fact that two groups arrived at the same result using different methods increases the likelihood that they have uncovered a significant phenomenon.

Although the association between the bacterium and colon cancer is highly suggestive, Holt cautioned that it was not enough to conclude that the relationship was causal. "Have you heard about Koch's postulates?" he asked. "Oh yes," I said, knowing by now that most investigators in this field found them exceedingly hard to fulfill. I recalled, "Barry Marshall had to drink an *H. pylori* cocktail to establish a causal connection." Holt said, laughing, "I don't think I'm prepared to do that. That's not even a little bit appealing. Barry Marshall was trying to satisfy Koch's postulates. Usually that's done in animal models but in this case

Barry Marshall *was* the animal model." Holt faces a similar dilemma; currently, he doesn't have an animal model.

Obviously more research needs to be done. If an animal model could be found or developed, that would help. A large cohort study could provide important information, but these take years to deliver results and are expensive. Holt said, "The next phase could take a long time. If we look at *H. pylori* as a model, we see that it took twenty years before causality was firmly established." This new approach to genomics doesn't answer all the questions, but at least it accelerates the identification of pathogens that are associated with cancer and that might be causal agents. Holt says he remains an "agnostic" about *Fusobacterium nucleatum*. Even if a causal relationship is not established, the fact that it is strongly linked to colon cancer could make it the basis of a diagnostic tool, much less invasive than a colonoscopy. Holt doesn't want to leap to conclusions, but his research has aroused much interest, in part because colon cancer is one of our most serious malignancies; in the US fifty thousand people die every year from colorectal cancer. Holt's discovery has the potential to save many lives. Numerous scientific journals and general interest publications reported on Holt and Myerson's work. The *New York Times* described the discoveries in an article called "Two Cancer Studies Find Bacterial Clue in Colon."[16]

YOU CAN *DO* SOMETHING ABOUT IT

So, can you catch cancer? Well, yes you can, although if Patrick Moore is right, you can't catch cancer from someone who has cancer. Nor is it likely that you would catch a *virus* from someone who has cancer. The vast majority of the time, cancer is a dead end for the pathogen. It no longer replicates. But you can catch a virus from someone in the earlier stages of an infection. And it might cause a cancer. So in that sense you can catch it.

Just as you can have epidemics of acute diseases, you can have cancer epidemics. Cancer of the liver, the cervix, and the stomach are all examples of malignancies that pathogens have spread throughout human populations. As Ludwik Gross intuited more than sixty years ago, for several reasons, scientists have had difficulty seeing those epidemics. The long lead time between the onset of infection and the development of symptoms obscured the relationship. More difficulties arose because with some viruses, such as HPV, you couldn't *see* the pathogenic agent at all. We needed new molecular tools to understand what was happening. The existence of cancer contagions has surprised both trained researchers and interested lay people. Palmer Beasley said, "These results shocked everyone. People wondered, 'How could the whole world have missed it? How could something that big have been sitting there?'" It leads one to speculate, as Robin Warren did, about what else we might be missing. Warren said, "There are probably things all around us that we're not seeing." The idea is both disconcerting and inspiring.

In *The Structure of Scientific Revolutions*, Thomas Kuhn observed that an accepted theory or paradigm does not fall because of a single counterexample. The old cancer paradigm is crumbling thanks to a score of discoveries. Each in their own unique way, the scientists I spoke to have helped to usher in a new medical era. The researchers took different paths, encountered different obstacles, and were endowed with different talents. Early on, Harald zur Hausen suspected that HPV was the cause of cervical cancer and spent ten years trying to prove it. Palmer Beasley, on the other hand, wasn't thinking of liver cancer at all when he stumbled across the evidence that hepatitis B caused it. His route to discovery was very different than zur Hausen's. Yet the investigators I interviewed had shared qualities and experiences too. Louis Pasteur didn't tell us what kind of preparation was necessary to make major scientific discoveries, but perhaps curiosity, a deep love of nature, and free-wheeling exploratory childhoods all have a role to play. Zur Hausen's mother boiled a fox skull for him—teeth and all. He kept it on his desk for years—for inspiration. Beasley's parents allowed him to amass a huge snake collection in suburban Los Angeles and his father even helped him to add to it on long starry nights in the Mojave Desert. Barry Marshall's parents let him wander around Kalgoorlie and didn't stop his experiments even after he singed his and his father's eyebrows a few times. Marshall said that Kalgoorlie formed him as someone who liked to "live dangerously." Daring helped create the change in thinking. The desire to nail *H. pylori* motivated Barry Marshall *and* his Kiwi colleague, Arthur Morris, to risk their own health by drinking *H. pylori* cocktails. Their miserable reaction to the colonizing bacteria was just what they needed to make an important point. Steadfast persistence played a part. These scientists often faced skepticism from their colleagues. Patrick Moore said "scorn and derision" greeted what he and Yuan Chang first discovered. Zur Hausen was dismayed when incredulous silence followed his suggestion that HPV might cause cervical cancer. Remarkably, a sympathetic interest from one or two individuals was often enough to keep them going. Recollecting the early days of his research, Robin Warren recounted, "In fact, there was only one doctor who did believe in what I was doing: my wife, Win, who was a psychiatrist, and who encouraged me." Serendipity contributed too. When *H. pylori* were neglected over an Easter weekend, they finally grew, showing that the bacteria could be cultured in the lab. There are no formulas for success, but an alert sensitivity to data can take you a long way. A "funny blue line" captured Warren's attention and set a research train in motion. A bad case of diarrhea started Paul Ewald asking new questions. And though these scientists might be described as "leading edge" because of the impact they have had on our future, they have also possessed a sharp historical sense. Zur Hausen paid attention to rare reports stretching back a hundred years; some doctors had seen genital warts turn malignant. He took note. Marshall read the careful observations of William Osler back in 1919. Though there was much that a physician like Osler didn't know—information that has been subsequently discovered—his power of observation was just as clear-eyed as that of any physician today. That's why history can inform medicine.

There are some things that don't seem to be necessary for remarkable discoveries. Good science, it appears, does not always start in prestigious and well-funded labs. When Barry Marshall and Robin Warren wrote their famous 1984 paper, neither were associated with a university or had backing from prestigious granting agencies. Marshall did not even have a permanent job! Yuan Chang started her search for a new virus with a modest grant of $15,000. Being an outstanding student did not seem to be so important either. Patrick Moore dropped out in eleventh grade, and though he was later accepted at university, it was not at an Ivy League school. Zur Hausen described himself as an "average" pupil in elementary school, and Ewald was a B-student in high school.

Though the idea of catching cancer sounds scary, it is actually a good thing. As Robert Holt said, "If you find a strong link to an infectious agent, you can *do* something about it." We can use antibiotics and vaccines to combat this disease. Vaccines are often credited with saving more lives than any other medical innovation; certainly they have eliminated smallpox and greatly reduced deaths from other illnesses such as polio, meningitis, and measles. We are starting to see widespread use of anti-cancer vaccines. Around the globe, almost a third of all newborns have received a vaccine which prevents hepatitis B—an intervention which reduces their risk of liver cancer by 70 percent.[17] Forty million women have been immunized against cervical cancer—up to now, the third-most common cancer among women. This is dramatically reducing cervical abnormalities that progress to cancer. Antibiotics too have saved countless lives. Stomach cancer rates in developed western countries are dropping and should continue to do so, in part due to declining rates of *H. pylori* infections.[18]

Zur Hausen is convinced we will detect more infectious causes of cancer and, thus, increase our ability to prevent it. Perhaps we can look forward to a day when we will no more fear cancer than we do polio or rubella. As our population ages and the burden of cancers grow, a better appreciation of what causes them and what might *prevent* a major portion of them comes at a most opportune time.

NOTES

INTRODUCTION

1. James T. Patterson, *The Dread Disease: Cancer and Modern American Culture* (Cambridge, Massachusetts: Harvard University Press, 1987).

1. MORE THAN A CURIOSITY

1. "An Inquiry into Certain Aspects of Eugene L. Opie," *Archives of Pathology* 34 (1942): I-6, as quoted by J. G. Kidd in "Stay as Close to Nature as You Can," *A Notable Career in Finding Out: Peyton Rous, 1879–1970* (New York: Rockefeller University Press, 1971), 34, http://books.google.ca/books?id=5iKe4UItndcC&printsec=frontcover&source=gbs_ge_summary_r&cad=0#v=onepage&q&f=false.

2. Ibid., 26.

3. Eva Becsei-Kilborn, "Scientific Discovery and Scientific Reputation: The Reception of Peyton Rous' Discovery of the Chicken Sarcoma Virus," *Journal of the History of Biology* 43, no. 1 (Spring 2010): 111–57, DOI: 10.1007/s10739-008-9171-y.

4. Francis Peyton Rous, "A Sarcoma of the Fowl Transmissible by an Agent Separable from the Tumor Cells," *Journal of Experimental Medicine* 13, no. 4 (April 1911): 400, http://jem.rupress.org/content/13/4/397.full.pdf+html.

5. Becsei-Kilborn, "Scientific Discovery and Scientific Reputation."

6. Ibid.

7. Ibid.

8. Ibid.

9. "Medicine: Cancer Virus," *Time Magazine*, March 18, 1946.
10. Ludwik Gross, "The Etiology of Leukemia: Recent Developments in the Studies of a Mouse Leukemia Virus," *Archives of Internal Medicine* 109, no. 4 (1962): 375, DOI: 10.1001/archinte.1962.03620160001001.
11. Denis Burkitt, "The Discovery of Burkitt's Lymphoma," *Cancer*, May 15, 1983, 1778.
12. Anthony M. Epstein, "The Origin of EBV Research: Discovery and Characterization of the Virus," in *Epstein-Barr Virus*, ed. Erle S. Robertson (Norfolk, UK: Caister Academic Press, 2005), 3.
13. Burkitt, "The Discovery of Burkitt's Lymphoma," 1779.
14. Denis Burkitt, "A Tumour Safari in East and Central Africa," *British Journal of Cancer* 15, no. 3 (September 1962): 380.
15. Burkitt, "The Discovery of Burkitt's Lymphoma," 1781.
16. Anthony M. Epstein, "The Origin of EBV Research," 6.
17. Ibid., 10.
18. Luther L. Terry, "The Surgeon General's First Report on Smoking and Health: A Challenge to the Medical Professions," in *The Cigarette Underworld*, ed. Alan Blum (Secaucus, NJ: Lyle Stuart, 1985), 15.
19. René Vallery-Radot, *The Life of Pasteur*, trans. R. L. Devonshire (New York: Doubleday, Page & Company, 1919), 76, http://archive.org/details/lifeofpasteur034972mbp .
20. "Breakaway: The Global Burden of Cancer—Challenges and Opportunities," Economist Intelligence Unit (2009), accessed August 28, 2012, http://www.livestrong.org/pdfs/GlobalEconomicImpact.

2. PALMER BEASLEY DISCOVERS A SILENT EPIDEMIC

1. "2000 Taiwanese Besiege Embassy," *Ocala Star Banner*, December 17, 1978, 8.
2. 1963 was still early days for American involvement in Vietnam. That year sixteen thousand military advisors were serving in Vietnam. But two years later, the number of Americans in the combat zone had grown more than tenfold.
3. W. Schaffner and M. F. LaForce, "Training Field Epidemiologists: Alexander D. Langmuir and the Epidemic Intelligence Service," *American Journal of Epidemiology* 144, no. 8 (1996): S17, http://aje.oxfordjournals.org/content/144/Supplement_8/S16.full.pdf.
4. Ron Falco and Sharon Israel Williams, *Waterborne Salmonella Outbreak in Alamosa, Colorado, March and April 2008*, Colorado Department of Health and the Environment, 2009.

5. Mark Pendergrast, *Inside the Outbreaks: The Elite Medical Detectives of the Epidemic Intelligence Service* (New York: Houghton Mifflin Harcourt, 2010), 48–49.

6. "Rubella and Congenital Malformations," *Lancet* 243, no. 6288 (March 1944): 316.

7. Baruch Blumberg, *Hepatitis B: The Hunt for a Killer Virus* (Princeton, NJ: Princeton University Press, 2002), 36–38.

8. Baruch Blumberg and Harvey J. Alter, "A 'New' Antigen in Leukemia Sera," *JAMA* 191 (1965): 543.

9. Blumberg, *Hepatitis B*, 120–2.

10. Irving Millman, Toby K. Eisenstein, and Baruch S. Blumberg, eds., *Hepatitis B: The Virus, the Disease, and the Vaccine* (New York: Plenum Press, 1984), 12.

11. Blumberg, *Hepatitis B*, 125.

12. R. Palmer Beasley, "Rocks along the Road to the Control of HBV and HCC," *Annals of Epidemiology* 19, no. 4 (2009): 231–34, DOI:10.1016/j.annepidem.2009.01.017.

13. C. E. Stevens, R. P. Beasley, Julia Tsui, et al., "Vertical Transmission of Hepatitis B Antigen in Taiwan," *New England Journal of Medicine* 292 (1975): 771–74.

14. Beasley, "Rocks along the Road," 232.

15. Ibid.

16. R. Palmer Beasley, "Development of Hepatitis B Vaccine," JAMA 302, no. 3 (July 2009): 322–24. DOI:10.1001/jama.2009.1024, http://jama.ama-assn.org/content/302/3/322.full.

17. R. Palmer Beasley, Chia-Chin Lin, Kwei-Yu Wang, et al., "Hepatitis B Immune Globulin (HBIG) Efficacy in the Interruption of Perinatal Transmission of Hepatitis B Virus Carrier Start," *Lancet*, August 22, 1981, 389.

18. George Chin-Yun Lee, Lu-Yu Hwang, R. Palmer Beasley, et al., "Immunogenicity of Hepatitis B Virus Vaccine in Healthy Chinese Neonates," *Journal of Infectious Diseases* 148, no. 3 (September 1983): 520.

19. "The Safety of Hepatitis B Vaccine Has Not Been Proved, Department of Health Disallows the Trial on Our Children," *Central Daily*, trans. Shih Be Winn, March 17, 1980.

20. Merck Sharp and Dohme, "Hepatitis B: Its Prevention by Vaccine," *Journal of Infectious Diseases* 143, no. 2 (February 1981): 301.

21. Ludwik Gross, "Is Cancer a Communicable Disease?" *Cancer Research* 4 (May 1944): 293–303, http://cancerres.aacrjournals.org/content/4/5/293.full.pdf.

22. Beasley, Lin, Wang, et al., "Hepatitis B Immune Globulin (HBIG) Efficacy," 388–93.

23. Like many other countries, Taiwan had both a president and a premier. The president was the head of state; the premier was responsible for actually running the country.

24. "Staff of American Institute in Taiwan (AIT) Accept Hepatitis B Vaccine, Confident of This Still Experimental Vaccine," *Central Daily*, trans. Shih Be Winn, February 19, 1981.

25. "Hepatitis Vaccine Is Permitted," *Central Daily*, trans. Shih Be Winn, February 20, 1981.

26. R. Palmer Beasley, George Chin-Yun Lee, Cheng-Hsiung Roan, et al., "Prevention of Perinatally Transmitted Hepatitis B Virus Infections with Hepatitis B Immune Globulin and Hepatitis B Vaccines," *Lancet*, November 12, 1983, 1099–1102.

27. M. H. Chang, C. J. Chen, M. S. Lai, "Universal Hepatitis B Vaccination in Taiwan and the Incidence of Hepatocellular Carcinoma in Children," *New England Journal of Medicine* 336 (June 26, 1997): 1855–59.

28. M. H. Chang, S. L. You, C. J. Chen, et al., "Decreased Incidence of Hepatocellular Carcinoma in Hepatitis B Vaccinees: A 20-year Follow-up Study," Journal of the National Cancer Institute 101, no. 19 (2009): 1348–55, DOI: 10.1093/jnci/djp288.

29. William Yardley, "R. Palmer Beasley, Expert on Hepatitis B, Dies at 76," *New York Times*, August 26, 2012, accessed August 29, 2012, http://www.nytimes.com/2012/08/27/us/r-palmer-beasley-hepatitis-b-researcher-dies-at-76.html.

30. M. Hu and Wen Chen, "Assessment of Total Economic Burden of Chronic Hepatitis B (CHB)-Related Diseases in Beijing and Guangzhou, China," *Value in Health* 12, Supplement 3 (2009): S89, http://download.journals.elsevierhealth.com/pdfs/journals/1098-3015/PIIS109830151060349X.pdf.

31. "Hepatitis B Fact Sheet," World Health Organization, July 2012, http://www.who.int/mediacentre/factsheets/fs204/en/.

3. HARALD ZUR HAUSEN SOLVES THE RIDDLE OF CERVICAL CANCER

1. William Rawls, W. A Tompkins, M. E. Figueroa, and J. L. Melnick, Herpesvirus Type Association with Carcinoma of the Cervix," *Science* 161, no. 3847 (September 20, 1968): 1255–56.

2. Harald zur Hausen and Katja Reuter, *Gegen Krebs: Die Geschichte Einer Provokativen Idee* (Reinbek bei Hamburg: Rowohlt Verlag GmbH, 2010), 115. The translation from the German is by Claudia Cornwall.

3. For a full list of participants, see *Cancer Research* 33 (June 1973): 1349, http://cancerres.aacrjournals.org/content/33/6/1349.full.pdf+html.

4. Today, in his eighties, Roizman is still an active researcher. In an April 2010 email, he wrote that he originally thought that latency would be easy and quick to understand. But "it turned out that I was wrong. We did not know enough about the virus to solve the riddle. . . . We are finally beginning to understand what is going on. The bottom line is that the little virus is very clever."

5. Clyde R. Goodheart, "Summary of Informal Discussion on General Aspects of Herpesviruses," *Cancer Research* 33 (June 1973): 1417–18, and zur Hausen and Reuter, *Gegen Krebs*, 116–17.

6. Harold M. Schmeck, Jr., "A New Virus Link with Cancer Seen; Scientists Find a Material That Could Start Disease," *New York Times*, November 11, 1972, 25.

7. Thomas Kuhn, *The Structure of Scientific Revolutions* (Chicago: University of Chicago Press, 1970), 64.

8. Harald zur Hausen, Heinrich Schulte-Holthausen, Hans Wolf, et al., "Attempts to Detect Virus-specific DNA in Human Tumors: II. Nucleic Acid Hybridizations with Complementary RNA of Human Herpes Group Viruses," *International Journal of Cancer* 13 (1974): 657–64, 42.

9. Harald zur Hausen, "*Condylomata Acuminata* and Human Genital Cancer," *Cancer Research* 36 (February 1976): 530.

10. Kuhn, *Structure of Scientific Revolutions*, 64.

11. Zur Hausen and Reuter, *Gegen Krebs*, 119.

12. A workaround was eventually developed using mice with defective immune systems. They don't reject transplants. They will accept human tissue and can then be used in experiments. But in 1972, this was not available to zur Hausen.

13. By the 1990s, the reason for this was discovered. HPV is adapted to growing in skin—a tissue which has layers of cells with different properties. In 1992, a scaffolding to mimic skin's architecture and grow HPV was created, but zur Hausen didn't have it. See C. Meyers, "Biosynthesis of Human Papillomavirus from a Continuous Cell Line upon Epithelial Differentiation," *Science* 257, no. 5072 (August 14, 1992): 971–73, DOI: 10.1126/science.1323879.

14. Harald zur Hausen, *Genome und Glaube: der Unsichbare Käfig* (Berlin: Springer Verlag, 2002).

15. M. E. Hankin, "The Bactericidal Action of the Waters of the Jamuna and Ganges Rivers on Cholera Microbes," *Annals d'Institut Pasteur* 10 (1896): 511–23.

16. Frederick W. Twort, "An Investigation on the Nature of Ultra-microscopic Viruses," *Lancet* 186, no. 4814 (1915): 1241–43, DOI : 10.1016/S0140-6736(01)20383-3.

17. David Shrayer, "Felix d'Herelle in Russia," *Bulletin de l'Institut Pasteur* 94 (1996): 91-96, DOI:10.1016/0020-2452(96)81737-4.

18. M. Felix d'Hérelle, "On an Invisible Microbe Antagonistic to Dysentery Bacilli," presented by M. Roux, *Comptes Rendus Academie des Sciences* 165 (1917): 373–75, DOI: 10.4161/bact.1.1.14941.

19. Felix d'Hérelle, *The Bacteriophage: Its Role in Immunity*, trans. George Smith (Baltimore, MD: Williams and Wilkins Co., 1922), 20–21, http://archive.org/stream/cu31924003218991#page/n5/mode/2up.

20. J. Bordet, "Le probleme de I'autolyse microbienne transmissible ou du bacteriophage," *Annals d'Institut Pasteur* 39 (1925): 711.

21. André Lwoff, "Nobel Lecture: Interaction among Virus, Cell, and Organism," August 29, 2012, http://www.nobelprize.org/nobel_prizes/medicine/laureates/1965/lwoff-lecture.html.

22. James Watson and Francis Crick, "The Molecular Structure of Nucleic Acids,"*Nature* 171 (1953): 737–38, http://www.nature.com/nature/dna50/watsoncrick.pdf.

23. Anthony M. Epstein, "The Origin of EBV Research: Discovery and Characterization of the Virus," in *Epstein-Barr Virus*, ed. Erle S. Robertson (Norfolk, UK: Caister Academic Press: 2005), 7.

24. Zur Hausen and Reuter, *Gegen Krebs*, 57.

25. Harald zur Hausen and Heinrich Schulte-Holthausen, "Presence of EB Virus Nucleic Acid Homology in a 'Virus-Free' Line of Burkitt Tumor Cells," *Nature* 227 (1970): 245–48.

26. Harald zur Hausen, "Viruses in Human Tumours—Reminiscences and Perspectives," *Cancer Research* 68 (1996): 8.

27. As quoted in zur Hausen and Reuter, *Gegen Krebs*, 175.

28. Ibid., 180.

29. Ibid., 181.

30. Matthias Dürst, L. Gissmann, H. Ikenberg, H. zur Hausen, et al., "A Papillomavirus DNA from a Cervical Carcinoma and Its Prevalence in Cancer Biopsy Samples from Different Geographical Regions," *Proceedings for the National Academy of Science* 80 (June 1983): 3812–15.

31. M. Dürst, L. Gissmann, H. Ikenberg, et al., "A New Type of Papillomavirus DNA, Its Presence in Genital Cancer Biopsies and Cell Lines Derived from Cervical Cancer," *EMBO Journal* 3 (1984): 1151–57.

32. Vladmir Vonka, J. Kanka, J. Jelínek, et al., "Prospective Study on Relationship between Cervical Neoplasia and Herpes Simplex Type 2 Virus. I.

Epidemiological Characteristics," *International Journal of Cancer* 33 (1984): 49–60.

33. Rebecca Skloot, *The Immortal Life of Henrietta Lacks* (New York: Random House, 2010).

34. Elisabeth Schwarz, U. K. Freese, L. Gissmann, et al., "Structure and Transcription of Human Papillomavirus Sequences in Cervical Carcinoma Cells," *Nature* 314 (March 7, 1985): 111–14, DOI: 10.1038/314111a0.

35. Magnus von Knebel Doeberitz, T. Oltersdorf, E. Schwarz, L. Gissmann, et al., "Correlation of Modified Human Papilloma Virus Early Gene Expression with Altered Growth Properties in C4-1 Cervical Carcinoma Cells," *Cancer Research* 48, no. 13 (1988): 3780–86.

36. Zur Hausen and Reuter, *Gegen Krebs*, 246.

37. Ibid., 247.

38. *IARC Monographs on the Evaluation of Carcinogenic Risks to Humans: Human Papillomaviruses*, vol. 64 (1995), http://monographs.iarc.fr/ENG/Monographs/vol64/volume64.pdf.

39. "FDA Licenses New Vaccine for Prevention of Cervical Cancer and Other Diseases in Females Caused by Human Papillomavirus," June 8, 2006, http://www.fda.gov/NewsEvents/Newsroom/PressAnnouncements/2006/ucm108666.htm.

4. BARRY MARSHALL, ROBIN WARREN, AND HELICOBACTER PYLORI

1. Norman Swan, "Dr. Robin Warren," Interviews with Australian Scientists, Australian Academy of Science, 2008, accessed August 29, 2012, http://www.science.org.au/scientists/interviews/w/rw.html.

2. Richard Whitehead, S. C. Truelove, and M. W. Gear, "The Histological Diagnosis of Chronic Gastritis in Fibreoptic Gastroscope Biopsy Specimens," *Journal of Clinical Pathology* 25 (1972): 1–11.

3. Robin Warren, "The Discovery of *Helicobacter pylori* in Perth, Western Australia," in *Helicobacter Pioneers: Firsthand Accounts from the Scientists Who Discovered Helicobacters, 1892–1982*, ed. Barry Marshall (Victoria, Australia: Blackwell Publishing, 2002), 155.

4. In 1945, Howard Florey received the Nobel Prize for Physiology and Medicine, together with Alexander Fleming and Ernst Chain—for their work in developing penicillin.

5. "J. Robin Warren—Autobiography," Nobelprize.org. July 28, 2012, http://www.nobelprize.org/nobel_prizes/medicine/laureates/2005/warren-autobio.html.

6. W. P. Fung, J. M. Papadimitriou, and L. R. Matz, "Endoscopic, Histological and Ultrastructural Correlations in Chronic Gastritis," *American Journal of Gastroenterology* 71 (1979): 269–79.

7. Warren, "The Discovery of *Helicobacter pylori*," 158.

8. Norman Swan, "Dr. Barry Marshall," Interviews with Australian Scientists, Australian Academy of Science, 2008, http://www.science.org.au/scientists/interviews/m/marshall.html.

9. Barry Marshall, "The Discovery That *Helicobacter pylori*, a Spiral Bacterium, Caused Peptic Ulcer Disease," in *Helicobacter Pioneers: Firsthand Accounts from the Scientists Who Discovered Helicobacters, 1892–1982*, ed. Barry Marshall (Victoria, Australia: Blackwell Publishing, 2002), 169.

10. Providing evidence that bacteria can withstand punishing conditions is just one of the interesting properties of these microbes, called *Thermus aquaticus*. Because of its heat-resistant properties, an enzyme found in *Thermus aquaticus* is used in polymerase chain reaction to replicate DNA.

11. Marshall, "The Discovery," 169.

12. Susummu Ito, "How I Discovered Helicobacters in Boston in 1967," in *Helicobacter Pioneers: Firsthand Accounts from the Scientists Who Discovered Helicobacters, 1892–1982*, ed. Barry Marshall (Victoria, Australia: Blackwell Publishing, 2002), 90.

13. A. Stone Freedberg, "An Early Study of Human Stomach Bacteria," in *Helicobacter Pioneers: Firsthand Accounts from the Scientists Who Discovered Helicobacters, 1892–1982*, ed. Barry Marshall (Victoria, Australia: Blackwell Publishing, 2002), 26.

14. E. D. Palmer, "Investigation of the Gastric Mucosa Spirochetes of the Human," *Gastroenterology* 27 (1954): 218–20.

15. Natale Figura and Laura Bianciardi, "Helicobacters Were Discovered in Italy in 1892: An Episode in the Scientific Life of an Eclectic Pathologist, Giulio Bizzozero," in *Helicobacter Pioneers: Firsthand Accounts from the Scientists Who Discovered Helicobacters, 1892–1982*, ed. Barry Marshall (Victoria, Australia: Blackwell Publishing, 2002), 1.

16. Encyclopaedia Britannica, 1962, s.v. "Gastric and Duodenal Ulcer."

17. Swan, "Dr. Barry Marshall."

18. B. J. Marshall and R. J. Warren, "Unidentified Curved Bacilli in the Stomachs of Patients with Gastritis and Peptic Ulceration," *Lancet* 323, no. 8390 (June 16, 1984): 1311–15, DOI: 10.1016/S0140-6736(84)91816-6.

19. Marshall, "The Discovery," 180.

20. Ibid., 184.

21. B. J. Marshall, "Unidentified Curved Bacilli on Gastric Epithelium in Active Chronic Gastritis," *Lancet* 323, no. 8388 (June 4, 1983): 1275.

22. A. D. Pearson, *Proceedings of the Second International Workshop on* Campylobacter *Infections, Brussels, 6–9 September 1983* (London: Public Health Laboratory Service, 1983), 5.

23. Terence Monmaney, "Marshall's Hunch," *New Yorker*, September 20, 1993, 65.

24. Marshall, "The Discovery," 189.

25. Marshall, "The Discovery," 193.

26. "Barry J. Marshall—Nobel Lecture: *Helicobacter* Connections," Nobelprize.org, July 29, 2012, http://www.nobelprize.org/nobel_prizes/medicine/laureates/2005/marshall-lecture.html.

27. Marshall and Warren, " Unidentified Curved Bacilli."

28. Marshall, "The Discovery," 196.

29. Lawrence K. Altman, "New Bacterium Linked to Painful Stomach Ills," *New York Times*, July 31, 1984, http://www.nytimes.com/1984/07/31/science/new-bacterium-linked-to-painful-stomach-ills.html?pagewanted=all.

30. B. J. Marshall, J. A. Armstrong, D. B. McGechie, et al., "Attempt to Fulfill Koch's Postulates for Pyloric *Campylobacter*," *Medical Journal of Australia* 142 (1985): 436.

31. Marshall, "The Discovery," 197.

32. Arthur J. Morris, M. Rafiq Ali, Gordon I. Nicholson, et al., "Long-term Follow-up of Voluntary Ingestion of *Helicobacter pylori*," *Annals of Internal Medicine* 114 (1991): 662–63.

33. Marshall, "The Discovery," 201.

34. "*Helicobacter pylori* in Peptic Ulcer Disease," NIH Consensus Statement 12, no. 1 (January 7–9, 1994): 1–23.

35. James Ewing, "The Relation of Gastric Ulcer to Cancer," *Annals of Surgery* 67, no. 6 (June 1918) : 723, http://www.ncbi.nlm.nih.gov/pmc/articles/PMC1426744/pdf/annsurg00759-0080.pdf.

36. David Forman, D. G.Newell, F. Fullerton, et al., "Association between Infection with *Helicobacter pylori* and Risk of Gastric Cancer: Evidence from a Prospective Investigation," *British Medical Journal* 302, no. 6788 (June 1, 1991): 1302–5.

37. A. Nomura, G. N. Stemmermann, P. H. Chyou, et al., "*Helicobacter pylori* Infection and Gastric Carcinoma in a Population of Japanese-Americans in Hawaii," *New England Journal of Medicine* 325 (1991): 1132–36.

38. Julie Parsonnet, Dan Vandersteen, Jeffrey Goates, et al., "*Helicobacter pylori* in Intestinal- and Diffuse-type Gastric Adenocarcinoma," *Journal of National Cancer Institute* 83 (1991): 640–43.

39. "Schistosomes, Liver Flukes and *Helicobacter pylori*," *IARC Monographs* 61 (1994): 220.

5. PAUL EWALD STALKS THE STEALTH INFECTIONS

1. Sievert Rohwer and Paul Ewald, "The Cost of Dominance and Advantage of Subordination in a Badge Signalling System," *Evolution* 35, no. 3 (1981): 441–54.

2. Paul W. Ewald, "Evolutionary Biology and the Treatment of Signs and Symptoms of Infectious Disease," *Journal of Theoretical Biology* 86 (1980): 169–76.

3. Paul W. Ewald, "Host-Parasite Relations, Vectors, and the Evolution of Disease Severity," *Annual Review of Ecology and Systematics* 14 (1983): 465–85.

4. Paul W. Ewald, "The Evolution of Virulence," *Scientific American*, April 1993, 88.

5. Paul W. Ewald, *Plague Time: How Stealth Infections Cause Cancers, Heart Disease, and Other Deadly Ailments* (New York: Simon and Schuster, 2000), 6.

6. Hippocrates, *On Airs, Waters, and Places*, trans. Francis Adams, Internet Classics Archive, http://classics.mit.edu//Hippocrates/airwatpl.html, accessed July 2012.

7. Gregory Cochran, Paul W. Ewald, Kyle D. Cochran, "Infectious Causation of Disease: An Evolutionary Perspective," *Perspectives in Biology and Medicine* 43, no. 3 (2000): 408.

8. Ewald, *Plague Time*, 43.

9. Siobhán M. O'Connor, C. E. Taylor, J. M. Hughes, et al., "Emerging Infectious Determinants of Chronic Diseases," *Emerging Infectious Diseases*, July 2006, DOI: 10.3201/eid1207.060037.

10. "What Is Chronic Disease?" Wise Geek, accessed July 2012, http://www.wisegeek.com/what-is-chronic-disease.htm.

11. *Global Status Report on Noncommunicable Diseases, 2010*, World Health Organization, vii, http://www.who.int/nmh/publications/ncd_report_full_en.pdf.

12. *Noncommunicable Diseases: Country Profiles, 2011*, World Health Organization, http://whqlibdoc.who.int/publications/2011/9789241502283_eng.pdf.

13. "10 Facts on Noncommunicable Diseases," World Health Organization, September 2011, accessed July 2012, http://www.who.int/features/factfiles/noncommunicable_diseases/en/index.html.

14. Lauren Sompayrac, *How Pathogenic Viruses Work* (Sudbury, MA: Jones and Bartlett Publishers, 2002), 54, 55.

15. Ewald, *Plague Time*, 6.

16. William Hamilton, "The Genetical Evolution of Social Behaviour I," *Journal of Theoretical Biology* 7, no. 1 (July 1964): 1–16, DOI: 10.1016/0022-5193(64)90038-4; and William Hamilton, "The Genetical Evolution of Social Behaviour II," *Journal of Theoretical Biology* 7, no. 1 (July 1964): 17–52, DOI: 10.1016/0022-5193(64)90039-6.

17. Joshua Lederberg, "J. B. S. Haldane (1949) on Infectious Disease and Evolution," *Genetics* 153 (September 1999): 1–3, http://www.ncbi.nlm.nih.gov/pmc/articles/PMC1460735/pdf/10471694.pdf.

18. Anthony C. Allison, "The Discovery of Resistance to Malaria of Sickle-Cell Heterozygotes," *Biochemistry and Molecular Biology Education* 30, no. 5 (September 2002): 279–87, DOI: 10.1002/bmb.2002.494030050108.

19. Ana Ferreira, Ivo Marguti, Ingo Bechmann, et al., "Sickle Hemoglobin Confers Tolerance to *Plasmodium* Infection," *Cell* 145, no. 3 (April 29, 2011): 398–409. DOI: 10.1016/j.cell.2011.03.049.

20. Ewald, *Plague Time*, 9.

21. Ibid., 63.

22. Cochran, Ewald, Cochran, "Infectious Causation of Disease," 417.

23. Kazuyuki Tanabe, Toshihiro Mita, Jombart Thibaut, et al., "*Plasmodium falciparum* Accompanied the Human Expansion out of Africa," *Current Biology* 20, no. 14 (June 2010): 1283–89.

24. Xin Yi, Yu Liang, Emilia Huerta-Sanchez, et al., "Sequencing of 50 Human Exomes Reveals Adaptation to High Altitude," *Science* 329, no. 5987 (July 2010): 75–78, DOI: 10.1126/science.1190371.

25. Anthony S. Gunnell, T. N. Tran, A. Torrång, et al., "Synergy between Cigarette Smoking and Human Papillomavirus Type 16 in Cervical Cancer *In situ* Development," *Cancer Epidemiology, Biomarkers & Prevention* 15 (November 2006): 2141–47; published online October 20, 2006; DOI: 10.1158/1055-9965.EPI-06-0399.

26. A. H. Allam, R. C. Thompson, L. S. Wann, et al., "Artherosclerosis in Ancient Egyptian Mummies: The Horus Story," *Journal of American College of Cardiology Imaging* 4, no. 4 (2011): 315–17, DOI: 10.1016/j.jcmg.2011.02.002.

27. Carlos Prates, Sandra Sousa, Carlos Oliveira, Salima Ikram, "Prostate Metastatic Bone Cancer in an Egyptian Ptolemaic Mummy, a Proposed Radiological Diagnosis," *International Journal of Paleopathology* 1–2 (October 2011): 98–103.

28. B. M. Rothschild, D. H. Tanke, M. Helbling II, et al., "Epidemiologic Study of Tumors in Dinosaurs," *Naturwissenschaften*, published online, October 2003, DOI: 10.1007/s00114-003-0473-9.

29. Cochran, Ewald, Cochran, "Infectious Causation of Disease," 419.

30. Sebastien Couraud, G. Zalcman, B. Milleron, et al., "Lung Cancer in Never Smokers—A Review," *European Journal of Cancer* 48, no. 9 (June 2012): 1299–1311. Published online March 28, 2012.

31. "What Is My Risk?" Lung Cancer Alliance, http://www.screenforlungcancer.org/what-is-my-risk/.

32. Paul Ewald and Holly Swain Ewald, *Controlling Cancer: A Powerful Plan for Taking On the World's Most Daunting Disease* (Kindle Single, TED Books: January 2012).

33. Eileen F. Dunne, Elizabeth R. Unger, Maya Sternberg, et al., "Prevalence of HPV Infection among Females in the United States," *JAMA* 297, no. 8 (February 28, 2007): 813–19.

34. Anna R. Giuliano, Ji-Hyun Lee, William Fulp, et al., "Incidence and Clearance of Genital Human Papillomavirus Infection in Men (HIM): A Cohort Study," *Lancet* 377, no. 9769 (March 12, 2011): 932–40, DOI: 10.1016/S0140-6736(10)62342-2.

35. Eileen M. Burd, "Human Papillomavirus and Cervical Cancer," *Clinical Microbiology Reviews* 16, no. 1 (January 2003): 1–17, http://www.ncbi.nlm.nih.gov/pmc/articles/PMC145302/

6. GENE HUNTERS

1. Yuan Chang, E. Cesarman, M. S. Pessin, et al., "Identification of Herpesvirus-like DNA Sequences in AIDS-associated Kaposi's Sarcoma," *Science* 265 (1994): 1865–69.

2. Lawrence K. Altman, "Going Off the Beaten Path to Track Down Clues about AIDS," *New York Times*, December 10, 1994, http://www.nytimes.com/1994/12/20/science/the-doctor-s-world-going-off-the-beaten-path-to-track-down-clues-about-aids.html.

3. Jon Cohen, "Is a New Virus the Cause of KS?" *Science* 266 (December 16, 1994): 1803.

4. V. Beral, T. A. Peterman, R. L. Berkelman, et al., "Kaposi's Sarcoma among Persons with AIDS: A Sexually Transmitted Infection?" *Lancet* 335, no. 8682 (1990): 123–28, DOI: 10.1016/0140-6736(90)90001-L .

5. N. Lisitsyn, N. Lisitsyn, Martin Wigler, "Cloning the Differences between Two Complex Genomes," *Science* 259 (1993): 946–51.

6. Jon Cohen, "Controversy: Is KS Really Caused by New Herpesvirus?" *Science* 268 (1995): 1847–48.

7. Ibid.

8. Shou-Jiang Gao, Lawrence Kingsley, Donald R. Hoover, et al., "Seroconversion to Antibodies against Kaposi's Sarcoma-associated Herpesvirus-re-

lated Latent Nuclear Antigens before the Development of Kaposi's Sarcoma," *New England Journal of Medicine* 335 (1996): 233–41.

9. "Researchers Confirm Herpesvirus Role in KS," *P&S Journal* 17, no. 1 (Winter 1997), http://www.cumc.columbia.edu/psjournal/archive/archives/jour_v17n1_0004.html.

10. "Biological Agents: A Review of Human Carcinogens," *IARC Monographs* 100B (2012): 195.

11. D. Max Parkin, F. Sitas, M. Chirenje, et al., "Part I: Cancer in Indigenous Africans—Burden, Distribution, and Trends," *Lancet Oncology* 9, no. 7 (July 2008): 683–92.

12. Huichen Feng, Masahiro Shuda, Yuan Chang, Patrick S. Moore, et al., "Clonal Integration of a Polyomavirus in Human Merkel Cell Carcinoma," *Science* 319 (February 22, 2008): 1096–1100, DOI: 10.1126/science.1151804.

13. "Agents Classified by the *IARC Monographs*, Volumes 1–105," accessed August 10, 2012, http://monographs.iarc.fr/ENG/Classification/ClassificationsCASOrder.pdf.

14. Alexander Swidsinksi, Y. Dörffel, V. Loening-Baucke, et al., "Acute Appendicitis Is Characterised by Local Invasion with *Fusobacterium nucleatum/necrophorum*," *Gut* 60, no. 1 (January 2011): 34–40. Published online November 18, 2009.

15. Mauro Castellarin, René L. Warren, J. Douglas Freeman, et al. "*Fusobacterium nucleatum* Infection Is Prevalent in Human Colorectal Carcinoma," *Genome Research*, October 18, 2011, DOI: 10.1101/gr.126516.111.

16. Gina Kolata, "Two Cancer Studies Find Bacterial Clue in Colon," *New York Times*, October 17, 2011, http://www.nytimes.com/2011/10/18/health/18cancer.html .

17. See chapter 2, note 28.

18. A. C. De Vries et al., "Epidemiological Trends of Pre-malignant Gastric Lesions; A Long-term Nationwide Study in the Netherlands," *Gut* 2007, DOI: 10.1136/gut.2007.127167.

BIBLIOGRAPHY

"10 Facts on Noncommunicable Diseases." World Health Organization. Accessed July 2012. http://www.who.int/features/factfiles/noncommunicable_diseases/en/index.html.

"2000 Taiwanese Besiege Embassy." *Ocala Star Banner*, December 17, 1978.

"Agents Classified by the *IARC Monographs*, Volumes 1–105." Accessed August 10, 2012. http://monographs.iarc.fr/ENG/Classification/ClassificationsCASOrder.pdf.

Allam, A. H., R. C. Thompson, L. S. Wann, et al. "Artherosclerosis in Ancient Egyptian Mummies: The Horus Story." *Journal of American College of Cardiology Imaging* 4, no. 4 (2011): 315–17. DOI: 10.1016/j.jcmg.2011.02.002.

Allison, Anthony C. "The Discovery of Resistance to Malaria of Sickle-Cell Heterozygotes." *Biochemistry and Molecular Biology Education* 30, no. 5 (September 2002): 279–87. DOI: 10.1002/bmb.2002.494030050108.

Altman, Lawrence K. "New Bacterium Linked to Painful Stomach Ills." *New York Times*, July 31, 1984. http://www.nytimes.com/1984/07/31/science/new-bacterium-linked-to-painful-stomach-ills.html?pagewanted=all.

Beasley, R. Palmer. "Development of Hepatitis B Vaccine." *JAMA* 302, no. 3 (July 2009): 322–24. DOI: 10.1001/jama.2009.1024. http://jama.ama-assn.org/content/302/3/322.full.

———. "Rocks along the Road to the Control of HBV and HCC." *Annals of Epidemiology* 19, no. 4 (2009): 231–34. DOI: 10.1016/j.annepidem.2009.01.017.

Beasley, R. Palmer, George Chin-Yun Lee, Cheng-Hsiung Roan, et al. "Prevention of Perinatally Transmitted Hepatitis B Virus Infections with Hepatitis B Immune Globulin and Hepatitis B Vaccines." *Lancet*, November 12, 1983.

Beasley, R. Palmer, Chia-Chin Lin, Kwei-Yu Wang, et al. "Hepatitis B Immune Globulin (HBIG) Efficacy in the Interruption of Perinatal Transmission of Hepatitis B Virus Carrier Start." *Lancet*, August 22, 1981: 388–93.

Becsei-Kilborn, Eva. "Scientific Discovery and Scientific Reputation: The Reception of Peyton Rous' Discovery of the Chicken Sarcoma Virus." *Journal of the History of Biology* 43, no. 1 (Spring 2010): 111–57. DOI: 10.1007/s10739-008-9171-y.

Beral, V., T. A. Peterman, R. L. Berkelman, et al. "Kaposi's Sarcoma among Persons with AIDS: A Sexually Transmitted Infection?" *Lancet* 335, no. 8682 (1990): 123–28. DOI: 10.1016/0140-6736(90)90001-L.

"Biological Agents: A Review of Human Carcinogens." *IARC Monographs* 100B (2012): 195.

Blumberg, Baruch. *Hepatitis B: The Hunt for a Killer Virus.* Princeton, NJ: Princeton University Press, 2002.

Blumberg, Baruch, and Harvey J. Alter. "A 'New' Antigen in Leukemia Sera." *JAMA* 191 (1965): 543.

Bordet, J. "Le probleme de l'autolyse microbienne transmissible ou du bacteriophage." *Annals d'Institut Pasteur* 39 (1925): 711.

"Breakaway: The Global Burden of Cancer—Challenges and Opportunities." Economist Intelligence Unit (2009). Accessed August 28, 2012. http://www.livestrong.org/pdfs/GlobalEconomicImpact.

Burkitt, Denis. "The Discovery of Burkitt's Lymphoma." *Cancer*, May 15, 1983.

———. "A Tumour Safari in East and Central Africa." *British Journal of Cancer* 15, no. 3 (September 1962): 380.

"Cancer Virus." *Time Magazine*, March 18, 1946.

Castellarin, Mauro, René L. Warren, J. Douglas Freeman, et al. "*Fusobacterium nucleatum* Infection Is Prevalent in Human Colorectal Carcinoma." *Genome Research*, October 18, 2011. DOI: 10.1101/gr.126516.111.

Chang, Mei-Hwei, San-Lin You, Chien-Jen Chen, et al. "Decreased Incidence of Hepatocellular Carcinoma in Hepatitis B Vaccinees: A 20-year Follow-up Study." *Journal of the National Cancer Institute* 101, no. 19 (2009): 1348–55. DOI: 10.1093/jnci/djp288.

Chang, M. H., C. J. Chen, M. S. Lai, et al. "Universal Hepatitis B Vaccination in Taiwan and the Incidence of Hepatocellular Carcinoma in Children." *New England Journal of Medicine* 336 (June 26, 1997): 1855–59.

Chang, Y., E. Cesarman, M. S. Pessin, et al. "Identification of Herpesvirus-like DNA Sequences in AIDS-associated Kaposi's Sarcoma." *Science* 265 (1994): 1865–69.

Cochran, Gregory, Paul W. Ewald, and Kyle D. Cochran. "Infectious Causation of Disease: An Evolutionary Perspective." *Perspectives in Biology and Medicine* 43, no. 3 (2000): 408.

Cohen, Jon. "Controversy: Is KS Really Caused by New Herpesvirus?" *Science* 268 (1995): 1847–48.

———. "Is a New Virus the Cause of KS?" *Science* 266 (December 16, 1994): 1803.

Couraud, S., G. Zalcman, B. Milleron, et al. "Lung Cancer in Never Smokers—A Review." *European Journal of Cancer* 48, no. 9 (June 2012): 1299–1311. Published online March 28, 2012.

De Vries, A. C., et al. "Epidemiological Trends of Pre-malignant Gastric Lesions; A Long-term Nationwide Study in the Netherlands." *Gut* 2007. DOI: 10.1136/gut.2007.127167.

d'Hérelle, M. Felix. *The Bacteriophage: Its Role in Immunity*. Trans. George Smith. Baltimore, MD: Williams and Wilkins Co., 1922. http://archive.org/stream/cu31924003218991#page/n5/mode/2up.

———. "On an Invisible Microbe Antagonistic to Dysentery Bacilli." Presented by M. Roux. *Comptes Rendus Academie des Sciences* 165 (1917): 373–75. DOI: 10.4161/bact.1.1.14941.

Dunne, Eileen F., Elizabeth R. Unger, Maya Sternberg, et al. "Prevalence of HPV Infection among Females in the United States." *JAMA* 297, no. 8 (February 28, 2007): 813–19.

Dürst, M., L. Gissmann, H. Ikenberg, and H. zur Hausen. "A Papillomavirus DNA from a Cervical Carcinoma and Its Prevalence in Cancer Biopsy Samples from Different Geographical Regions." *Proceedings for the National Academy of Science* 80 (June 1983): 3812–15.

Dürst, M., L. Gissmann, H. Ikenberg, et al. "A New Type of Papillomavirus DNA, Its Presence in Genital Cancer Biopsies and Cell Lines Derived from Cervical Cancer." *EMBO Journal* 3 (1984): 1151–57.

Epstein, Anthony M. "The Origin of EBV Research: Discovery and Characterization of the Virus." In *Epstein-Barr Virus*, edited by Erle S. Robertson. Norfolk, UK: Caister Academic Press, 2005.

Ewald, Paul W. "The Evolution of Virulence." *Scientific American*, April 1993.

———. "Evolutionary Biology and the Treatment of Signs and Symptoms of Infectious Disease." *Journal of Theoretical Biology* 86 (1980): 169–76.

———. "Host-Parasite Relations, Vectors, and the Evolution of Disease Severity." *Annual Review of Ecology and Systematics* 14 (1983): 465–85.

———. *Plague Time: How Stealth Infections Cause Cancers, Heart Disease, and Other Deadly Ailments*. New York: Simon and Schuster, 2000.

Ewald, Paul, and Holly Swain Ewald. *Controlling Cancer: A Powerful Plan for Taking On the World's Most Daunting Disease*. Kindle Single, TED Books, January 2012.

Ewing, James. "The Relation of Gastric Ulcer to Cancer." *Annals of Surgery* 67, no. 6 (June 1918): 723. http://www.ncbi.nlm.nih.gov/pmc/articles/PMC1426744/pdf/annsurg00759-0080.pdf.

Falco, Ron, and Sharon Israel Williams. *Waterborne* Salmonella *Outbreak in Alamosa Colorado, March and April 2008*. Colorado Department of Health and the Environment, 2009. Accessed August 28, 2012. http://www.cdphe.state.co.us/wq/drinkingwater/pdf/AlamosaInvestRpt.pdf.

"FDA Licenses New Vaccine for Prevention of Cervical Cancer and Other Diseases in Females Caused by Human Papillomavirus." June 8, 2006. http://www.fda.gov/NewsEvents/Newsroom/PressAnnouncements/2006/ucm108666.htm.

Feng, Huichen, Masahiro Shuda, Yuan Chang, Patrick S. Moore. "Clonal Integration of a Polyomavirus in Human Merkel Cell Carcinoma." *Science* 319 (February 22, 2008): 1096–1100. DOI: 10.1126/science.1151804.

Ferreira, Ana, Ivo Marguti, Ingo Bechmann, et al. "Sickle Hemoglobin Confers Tolerance to *Plasmodium* Infection." *Cell* 145, no. 3 (April 29, 2011): 398–409, 29. DOI: 10.1016/j.cell.2011.03.049.

Figura, Natale, and Laura Bianciardi. "Helicobacters Were Discovered in Italy in 1892: An Episode in the Scientific Life of an Eclectic Pathologist, Giulio Bizzozero." In *Helicobacter Pioneers: Firsthand Accounts from the Scientists Who Discovered Helicobacters, 1892–1982*, edited by Barry Marshall. Victoria, Australia: Blackwell Publishing, 2002.

Forman, D., D. G. Newell, F. Fullerton, et al. "Association between Infection with *Helicobacter pylori* and Risk of Gastric Cancer: Evidence from a Prospective Investigation." *British Medical Journal* 302, no. 6788 (June 1, 1991): 1302–5.

Freedberg, A. Stone. "An Early Study of Human Stomach Bacteria." In *Helicobacter Pioneers: Firsthand Accounts from the Scientists Who Discovered Helicobacters, 1892–1982*, edited by Barry Marshall. Victoria, Australia: Blackwell Publishing, 2002.

Fung, W. P., J. M. Papadimitriou, L. R. Matz. "Endoscopic, Histological and Ultrastructural Correlations in Chronic Gastritis." *American Journal of Gastroenterology* 71 (1979): 269–79.

Gao, Shou-Jiang, Lawrence Kingsley, Donald R. Hoover, et al. "Seroconversion to Antibodies against Kaposi's Sarcoma-associated Herpesvirus-related Latent Nuclear Antigens before the Development of Kaposi's Sarcoma." *New England Journal of Medicine* 335 (1996): 233–41.

Giuliano, Anna R., Ji-Hyun Lee, William Fulp, et al. "Incidence and Clearance of Genital Human Papillomavirus Infection in Men (HIM): A Cohort Study," *Lancet* 377, no. 9769 (March 12, 2011): 932–40. DOI: 10.1016/S0140-6736(10)62342-2.

Global Status Report on Noncommunicable Diseases, 2010. World Health Organization. http://www.who.int/nmh/publications/ncd_report_full_en.pdf.

Goodheart, Clyde R. " Summary of Informal Discussion on General Aspects of Herpesviruses." *Cancer Research* 33 (June 1973): 1417–18.

Gross, Ludwik. "The Etiology of Leukemia: Recent Developments in the Studies of a Mouse Leukemia Virus." *Archives of Internal Medicine* 109, no. 4 (1962): 375. DOI: 10.1001/archinte.1962.03620160001001.

———. "Is Cancer a Communicable Disease?" *Cancer Research* 4 (May 1944): 293–303. http://cancerres.aacrjournals.org/content/4/5/293.full.pdf.

Gunnell, A. S., T. N. Tran, A. Torrång, et al. "Synergy between Cigarette Smoking and Human Papillomavirus Type 16 in Cervical Cancer *In situ* Development," *Cancer Epidemiology, Biomarkers & Prevention* 15 (November 2006): 2141–47. Published online October 20, 2006. DOI: 10.1158/1055-9965.EPI-06-0399.

Hamilton, William. "The Genetical Evolution of Social Behaviour I." *Journal of Theoretical Biology* 7, no. 1 (July 1964): 1–16. DOI: 10.1016/0022-5193(64)90038-4.

———. "The Genetical Evolution of Social Behaviour II." *Journal of Theoretical Biology* 7, no. 1 (July 1964): 17–52. DOI: 10.1016/0022-5193(64)90039-6.

Hankin, M. E. "The Bactericidal Action of the Waters of the Jamuna and Ganges Rivers on Cholera Microbes." *Annals d'Institut Pasteur* 10 (1896): 511–23.

"*Helicobacter pylori* in Peptic Ulcer Disease." NIH Consensus Statement 12, no. 1 (January 7–9, 1994): 1–23.

"Hepatitis B Fact Sheet." World Health Organization. July 2012. http://www.who.int/mediacentre/factsheets/fs204/en/.

"Hepatitis Vaccine Is Permitted." *Central Daily*. Trans. Shih Be Winn. February 20, 1981.

Hippocrates. *On Airs, Waters, and Places*. Trans. Francis Adams, Internet Classics Archive. Accessed July 2012. http://classics.mit.edu//Hippocrates/airwatpl.html.

Hu, M., and W. Chen. "Assessment of Total Economic Burden of Chronic Hepatitis B (CHB)–Related Diseases in Beijing and Guangzhou, China." *Value in Health* 12, supplement 3 (2009): S89. http://download.journals.elsevierhealth.com/pdfs/journals/1098-3015/PIIS109830151060349X.pdf.

IARC Monographs on the Evaluation of Carcinogenic Risks to Humans: *Human Papillomaviruses*. Vol. 64 (1995). http://monographs.iarc.fr/ENG/Monographs/vol64/volume64.pdf.

Ito, Susummu. "How I Discovered Helicobacters in Boston in 1967." In *Helicobacter Pioneers: Firsthand Accounts from the Scientists Who Discovered Helicobacters, 1892–1982*, edited by Barry Marshall. Victoria, Australia: Blackwell Publishing, 2002.

Kidd, J. G. "Stay As Close to Nature As You Can." In *A Notable Career in Finding Out: Peyton Rous, 1879–1970*. New York: Rockefeller University Press, 1971.

Kolata, Gina. "Two Cancer Studies Find Bacterial Clue in Colon." *New York Times*, October 17, 2011. http://www.nytimes.com/2011/10/18/health/18cancer.html.

Kuhn, Thomas. *The Structure of Scientific Revolutions*. Chicago: University of Chicago Press, 1970.

Lederberg, Joshua. "J. B. S. Haldane (1949) on Infectious Disease and Evolution." *Genetics* 153 (September 1999): 1–3. http://www.ncbi.nlm.nih.gov/pmc/articles/PMC1460735/pdf/10471694.pdf.

Lee, George Chin-Yun, Lu-Yu Hwang, R. Palmer Beasley, et al. "Immunogenicity of Hepatitis B Virus Vaccine in Healthy Chinese Neonates." *Journal of Infectious Diseases* 148, no. 3 (September 1983): 520.

Lisitsyn N., N. Lisitsyn, M. Wigler. "Cloning the Differences between Two Complex Genomes." *Science* 259 (1993): 946–51.

List of Participants. *Cancer Research* 33 (June 1973): 1349. http://cancerres.aacrjournals.org/content/33/6/1349.full.pdf+html.

Luther, L. Terry. "The Surgeon General's First Report on Smoking and Health: A Challenge to the Medical Professions." In *Cigarette Underworld*, edited by Alan Blum. Secaucus, NJ: Lyle Stuart, 1985.

Lwoff, André. "Nobel Lecture: Interaction among Virus, Cell, and Organism." August 29, 2012. http://www.nobelprize.org/nobel_prizes/medicine/laureates/1965/lwoff-lecture.html.

Marshall, Barry. "The Discovery That *Helicobacter pylori*, a Spiral Bacterium, Caused Peptic Ulcer Disease." In *Helicobacter Pioneers: Firsthand Accounts from the Scientists Who Discovered Helicobacters, 1892–1982*, edited by Barry Marshall. Victoria, Australia: Blackwell Publishing, 2002.

———. "Nobel Lecture: *Helicobacter* Connections." Nobelprize.org. July 29, 2012. http://www.nobelprize.org/nobel_prizes/medicine/laureates/2005/marshall-lecture.html.

Marshall, B. J., J. A. Armstrong, D. B. McGechie, R. J. Glancy. "Attempt to Fulfill Koch's Postulates for Pyloric *Campylobacter*." *Medical Journal of Australia* 142 (1985): 436.

Marshall, B. J., and R. J. Warren. "Unidentified Curved Bacilli in the Stomachs of Patients with Gastritis and Peptic Ulceration." *Lancet* 323, no. 8390 (June 16, 1984): 1311–15.

McIntosh, Noel. "Human Papilloma Virus and Cervical Cancer." *Reproductive Health Online*. An affiliate of Johns Hopkins University. Accessed September 1, 2012. http://www.reproline.jhu.edu/english/3cc/3refman/cxca_hpv1.htm.

Merck Sharp and Dohme. "Hepatitis B: Its Prevention by Vaccine." *Journal of Infectious Diseases* 143, no. 2 (February 1981): 301.

Meyers, C. "Biosynthesis of Human Papillomavirus from a Continuous Cell Line upon Epithelial Differentiation." *Science* 257, no. 5072 (August 14, 1992): 971–73. DOI: 10.1126/science.1323879.

Millman, Irving, Toby K. Eisenstein, Baruch Blumberg, eds. *Hepatitis B: The Virus, the Disease, and the Vaccine*. New York: Plenum Press, 1984.

Monmaney, Terrence. "Marshall's Hunch." *New Yorker*, September 20, 1993.

Morris, Arthur J., M. Rafiq Ali, Gordon I. Nicholson, et al. "Long-Term Follow-up of Voluntary Ingestion of *Helicobacter pylori*." *Annals of Internal Medicine* 114 (1991): 662–63.

Nomura, A., G. N. Stemmermann, P. H. Chyou, et al. "*Helicobacter pylori* Infection and Gastric Carcinoma in a Population of Japanese-Americans in Hawaii." *New England Journal of Medicine* 325 (1991): 1132–36.

Noncommunicable Diseases: Country Profiles, 2011. World Health Organization. http://whqlibdoc.who.int/publications/2011/9789241502283_eng.pdf.

O'Connor, S. M., C. E. Taylor, J. M. Hughes. "Emerging Infectious Determinants of Chronic Diseases." *Emerging Infectious Diseases*, July 2006. DOI: 10.3201/eid1207.060037.

Palmer, E. D. "Investigation of the Gastric Mucosa Spirochetes of the Human." *Gastroenterology* 27 (1954): 218–20.

Parkin, D. M., F. Sitas, M. Chirenje, et al. "Part I: Cancer in Indigenous Africans—Burden, Distribution, and Trends." *Lancet Oncology* 9, no. 7 (July 2008): 683–92.

Parsonnet, Julie, Dan Vandersteen, Jeffrey Goates, et al. "*Helicobacter pylori* in Intestinal- and Diffuse-type Gastric Adenocarcinoma." *Journal of the National Cancer Institute* 83 (1991): 640–43.

Patterson, James T. *The Dread Disease: Cancer and Modern American Culture*. Cambridge, MA: Harvard University Press, 1987.

Pearson, A. D. *Proceedings of the Second International Workshop on* Campylobacter *Infections, Brussels, 6–9 September 1983*. London: Public Health Laboratory Service, 1983.

Pendergrast, Mark. *Inside the Outbreaks: The Elite Medical Detectives of the Epidemic Intelligence Service*. New York: Houghton Mifflin Harcourt, 2010.

Peyton Rous, Francis. "A Sarcoma of the Fowl Transmissible by an Agent Separable from the Tumor Cells." *Journal of Experimental Medicine* 13, no. 4 (April 1911): 400. http://www.jem.org/cgi/reprint/13/4/397.

Prates, Carlos, Sandra Sousa, Carlos Oliveira, Salima Ikram. "Prostate Metastatic Bone Cancer in an Egyptian Ptolemaic Mummy, a Proposed Radiological Diagnosis." *International Journal of Paleopathology* 1–2 (October 2011): 98–103.

Rawls, W. E., W. A. Tompkins, M. E. Figueroa, J. L. Melnick. "Herpesvirus Type 2: Association with Carcinoma of the Cervix." *Science* 161, no. 3847 (September 20, 1968): 1255–56.

"Researchers Confirm Herpesvirus Role in KS." *P&S Journal* 17, no. 1 (Winter 1997). http://www.cumc.columbia.edu/psjournal/archive/archives/jour_v17n1_0004.html.

Rohwer, Sievert, and Paul Ewald. "The Cost of Dominance and Advantage of Subordination in a Badge Signalling System." *Evolution* 35, no. 3 (1981): 441–54.

Rothschild, B. M., D. H. Tanke, M. Helbling II, et al. "Epidemiologic Study of Tumors in Dinosaurs." *Naturwissenschaften*. Published online, October 2003. DOI: 10.1007/s00114-003-0473-9.

"Rubella and Congenital Malformations." *Lancet* 243, no. 6288 (March 1944): 316.

"The Safety of Hepatitis B Vaccine Has Not Been Proved, Department of Health Disallows the Trial on Our Children." Trans. Shih Be Winn. *Central Daily*. March 17, 1980.

Schaffner, W., and M. F. LaForce. "Training Field Epidemiologists: Alexander D. Langmuir and the Epidemic Intelligence Service." *American Journal of Epidemiology* 144, no. 8 (1996): S17. http://aje.oxfordjournals.org/content/144/Supplement_8/S16.full.pdf.

"Schistosomes, Liver Flukes and *Helicobacter pylori*." *IARC Monographs* 61 (1994): 220.

Schmeck, Harold M., Jr. "A New Virus Link with Cancer Seen; Scientists Find a Material That Could Start Disease." *New York Times*, November 11, 1972, 25.

Schwarz, E., U. K. Freese, L. Gissmann, et al. "Structure and Transcription of Human Papillomavirus Sequences in Cervical Carcinoma Cells." *Nature* 314 (March 7, 1985): 111–14. DOI: 10.1038/314111a0.

Shrayer, David. "Felix d'Herelle in Russia," *Bulletin de l'Institut Pasteur* 94 (1996): 91–96. DOI:10.1016/0020-2452(96)81737-4.

Skloot, Rebecca. *The Immortal Life of Henrietta Lacks*. New York: Random House, 2010.

Sompayrac, Lauren. *How Pathogenic Viruses Work*. Sudbury, MA: Jones and Bartlett Publishers, 2002.

"Staff of American Institute in Taiwan (AIT) Accept Hepatitis B Vaccine, Confident of This Still Experimental Vaccine." *Central Daily*. Trans. Shih Be Winn. February 19, 1981.

Stevens, Cladd E., R. Palmer Beasley, et al. "Vertical Transmission of Hepatitis B Antigen in Taiwan." *New England Journal of Medicine* 292 (1975): 771–74.

Swan, Norman. "Dr. Barry Marshall." Interviews with Australian Scientists. Australian Academy of Science, 2008. http://www.science.org.au/scientists/interviews/m/marshall.html.

———. "Dr. Robin Warren." Interviews with Australian Scientists. Australian Academy of Science, 2008. http://www.science.org.au/scientists/interviews/m/marshall.html.

Swidsinksi, Alexander, Y. Dörffel, V. Loening-Baucke, et al. "Acute Appendicitis Is Characterised by Local Invasion with *Fusobacterium nucleatum/necrophorum*." *Gut* 60, no. 1 (January 2011): 34–40. Published online November 18, 2009.

Tanabe, Kazuyuki, Toshihiro Mita, Thibaut Jombart, et al. "*Plasmodium falciparum* Accompanied the Human Expansion out of Africa." *Current Biology* 20, no. 14 (June 2010): 1283–89.

Twort, Frederick W. "An Investigation on the Nature of Ultra-microscopic Viruses." *Lancet* 186, no. 4814 (1915): 1241–43. DOI: 10.1016/S0140-6736(01)20383-3.

Vallery-Radot, René. *The Life of Pasteur*. Trans. R. L. Devonshire. New York: Doubleday, Page & Company, 1919. http://archive.org/details/lifeofpasteur034972mbp.

Vonka, V., J. Kanka, J. Jelínek, et al. "Prospective Study on Relationship between Cervical Neoplasia and Herpes Simplex Type 2 Virus. I. Epidemiological Characteristics." *International Journal of Cancer* 33 (1984): 49–60.

von Knebel Doeberitz, M., T. Oltersdorf, E. Schwarz, L. Gissmann. "Correlation of Modified Human Papilloma Virus Early Gene Expression with Altered Growth Properties in C4-1 Cervical Carcinoma Cells." *Cancer Research* 48, no. 13 (1988): 3780–86.

Warren, J. Robin. "Autobiography." Nobelprize.org. July 28, 2012. http://www.nobelprize.org/nobel_prizes/medicine/laureates/2005/warren-autobio.html.

———. "The Discovery of *Helicobacter pylori* in Perth, Western Australia." In *Helicobacter Pioneers: Firsthand Accounts from the Scientists Who Discovered Helicobacters, 1892–1982*, edited by Barry Marshall. Victoria, Australia: Blackwell Publishing, 2002.

Warren, Robin, and Barry Marshall. "Unidentified Curved Bacilli in the Stomach of Patients with Gastritis and Peptic Ulceration." *Lancet* 1, no. 8390 (1984): 1311–15. DOI: 10.1016/S0140-6736(84)91816-6.

———. "Unidentified Curved Bacilli on Gastric Epithelium in Active Chronic Gastritis." *Lancet* 323, no. 8388 (June 4, 1983): 1275.

Watson, James, and Francis Crick. "The Molecular Structure of Nucleic Acids."*Nature* 171 (1953): 737–38. http://www.nature.com/nature/dna50/watsoncrick.pdf.

Weber, G., J. Shendure, D. M. Tanenbaum, et al. "Identification of Foreign Gene Sequences by Transcript Filtering against the Human Genome." *Nature Genetics* 2, no. 141 (February 2002): 2. Published online January 14, 2002.

"What Is Chronic Disease?" Wise Geek. Accessed July 2012. http://www.wisegeek.com/what-is-chronic-disease.htm.

"What Is My Risk?" Lung Cancer Alliance. http://www.screenforlungcancer.org/what-is-my-risk/.

Whitehead, R., S. C. Truelove, M. W. Gear. "The Histological Diagnosis of Chronic Gastritis in Fibreoptic Gastroscope Biopsy Specimens." *Journal of Clinical Pathology* 25 (1972): 1–11.

Yardley, William. "R. Palmer Beasley, Expert on Hepatitis B, Dies at 76." *New York Times*, August, 26, 2012. Accessed August 29, 2012. http://www.nytimes.com/2012/08/27/us/r-palmer-beasley-hepatitis-b-researcher-dies-at-76.html.

Yi, Xin, Yu Liang, Emilia Huerta-Sanchez, et al. " Sequencing of 50 Human Exomes Reveals Adaptation to High Altitude." *Science* 329, no. 5987 (July 2010): 75–78. DOI: 10.1126/science.1190371.

zur Hausen, Harald. "*Condylomata acuminata* and Human Genital Cancer." *Cancer Research 36* (February 1976): 530.

———. *Genome und Glaube: der Unsichbare Käfig*. Berlin: Springer Verlag, 2002.

———."Viruses in Human Tumours—Reminiscences and Perspectives." *Cancer Research* 68 (1996): 8.

zur Hausen, Harald, and Katja Reuter. *Gegen Krebs: Die Geschichte Einer Provokativen Idee*. Reinbek bei Hamburg: Rowohlt Verlag GmbH, 2010.

zur Hausen, H., and H. Schulte-Holthausen. "Presence of EB Virus Nucleic Acid Homology in a 'Virus-free' Line of Burkitt Tumor Cells." *Nature* 227 (1970): 245–48.

zur Hausen, Harald, Heinrich Schulte-Holthausen, Hans Wolf, et al. "Attempts to Detect Virus-specific DNA in Human Tumors: II. Nucleic Acid Hybridizations with Complementary RNA of Human Herpes Group Viruses." *International Journal of Cancer* 13 (1974): 657–64, 42.

INDEX

ABOUT THE AUTHOR

Claudia Cornwall was born in Shanghai, and came to Canada with her parents when she was nearly a year old. She studied philosophy at the University of British Columbia and obtained a PhD in philosophy from the University of Calgary. Her thesis looked at whether or not sign-language-using chimps were genuine language users.

Cornwall has been a freelance journalist for nearly thirty years. She is curious about many subjects, but medicine has been an abiding interest. She has written four books and over fifty articles for general interest magazines, many on medical and health issues. She wrote a popular yearly feature for *Reader's Digest Canada* on medical breakthroughs. Her recent book, , was a finalist for the 2012 Vancouver Book Award. A memoir, *Letter from Vienna: A Daughter Uncovers Her Family's Jewish Past* won the BC Prize for Best Non-Fiction in 1996. Cornwall has also received several writing grants; most recently, a $20,000 award from the Canadian Institutes of Health to support her work on *Catching Cancer*. She teaches courses on creative writing and on legal and ethical issues for writers at Simon Fraser University and Douglas College. She lives in Vancouver with her husband, Gordon Cornwall, and her cat, a Maine Coon. She has two children in their twenties.